PocketRadiologist™
Spine
Top 100 Diagnoses

PocketRadiologist™
Spine
100 Top Diagnoses

Michael Brant-Zawadzki MD FACR
Medical Director, Department of Radiology
Hoag Memorial Hospital
Newport Beach, California

Mark Z Chen MD
Department of Radiology
Hoag Memorial Hospital
Newport Beach, California

Kevin R Moore, MD
Assistant Professor of Radiology
Section of Neuroradiology
Residency Program Director
University of Utah School of Medicine
Salt Lake City, Utah

Karen L Salzman MD
Assistant Professor of Radiology
Section of Neuroradiology
University of Utah School of Medicine
Salt Lake City, Utah

Anne G Osborn MD FACR
University Distinguished Professor of Radiology
William H and Patricia W Child Presidential Endowed Chairholder
University of Utah School of Medicine
Salt Lake City, Utah

Amersham Health Visiting Professor in Diagnostic Imaging
Armed Forces Institute of Pathology
Washington, DC

With 200 drawings and radiographic images

Drawings: *James A Cooper MD*
              Walter Stuart MFA
              Lane R Bennion MS

Image Editing: *Ming Q Huang MD*
               Melissa Petersen

AMIRSYS™

W. B. SAUNDERS COMPANY
An Elsevier Science Company

AMIRSYS™

A medical reference publishing company

First Edition

Text - Copyright Michael Brant-Zawadzki 2002

Drawings - Copyright Amirsys Inc 2002

Compilation - Copyright Amirsys Inc 2002

First Printing: April 2002
Second Printing: October 2002

Composition by Amirsys Inc, Salt Lake City, Utah

Printed by K/P Corporation, Salt Lake City, Utah

ISBN: 0-7216-0675-X

Preface

The **PocketRadiologist™** series is an innovative, quick reference designed to deliver succinct, up-to-date information to practicing professionals "at the point of service." As close as your pocket, each title in the series is written by world-renowned authors, specialists in their area. These experts have designated the "top 100" diagnoses in every major body area, bulleted the most essential facts, and offered high-resolution imaging to illustrate each topic. Selected references are included for further review. Full color anatomic-pathologic computer graphics model many of the actual diseases.

Each **PocketRadiologist™** title follows an identical format. The same information is in the same place—every time—and takes you quickly from key facts to imaging findings, differential diagnosis, pathology, pathophysiology, and relevant clinical information.

PocketRadiologist™ titles are available in both print and hand-held PDA formats. Our first modules feature Spine, Head and Neck, and Orthopedic (Musculoskeletal) Imaging. Additional titles include Spine and Cord, Chest, Breast, Vascular, Cardiac, Pediatrics, Emergency, and Genital Urinary, and Gastro Intestinal. Enjoy!

Anne G Osborn MD
Editor-in-Chief, Amirsys Inc

Notice and Disclaimer

PocketRadiologist™
Spine
Top 100 Diagnoses

The diagnoses in this book are divided into 11 sections in the following order:

Congenital
Trauma
Degenerative
Infections
Inflammatory/Autoimmune
Neoplasms
Non-Neoplastic Cysts and Masses
Post Operative Complications
Vascular Lesions
Vertebral Marrow Changes
Peripheral Nerve/Plexus Imaging

Table of Diagnoses

Congenital

Trauma

Degenerative

Infections

Inflammatory / Autoimmune

Neoplasms

Non-Neoplastic Cysts and Masses

Post Operative Complications

CONGENITAL

Neurenteric Cyst

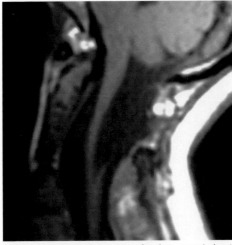

Sagittal T1WI of the cervical spine demonstrates fused upper cervical vertebral bodies. There is a capacious fluid-filled space in the posterior upper cervical canal.

Key Facts
- Synonym: Enterogenous cyst
- Definition: Intraspinal enteric-lined cyst
- Classic imaging appearance: Intradural extramedullary cyst with associated vertebral anomalies
- Other key facts
  - Along the spectrum of split notochord syndrome
  - Most common in the anterior thoracic (42% in one series) or cervical spine (32%), rare in lumbar spine
  - Usually midline
  - Vertebral anomalies including spina bifida, vertebral fusion, butterfly vertebra, or scoliosis in about half of the cases

Imaging Findings
General Features
- Best imaging clue: Vertebral anomalies with an intraspinal cyst
CT Myelogram Findings
- Vertebral anomalies
- Focal enlargement of the canal
- Intradural extramedullary cyst
- Invaginating cyst may mimic an intramedullary lesion
MR Findings
- Well-circumscribed, intradural, extramedullary fluid-intensity lesion
  - Iso- to hyperintense to cerebral spinal fluid (CSF) on T1WI and T2WI depending on protein content
  - No enhancement after contrast injection
  - Focal cord atrophy from chronic mass effect
Imaging Recommendations
- Coronal T1WI to better assess vertebral anomalies

Neurenteric Cyst

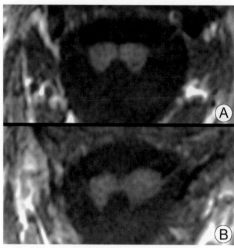

Axial T1WI (A, B) of the upper cervical spine reveals a cyst isointense to CSF, splaying the posterior cervical cord at the midline.

Differential Diagnosis

Arachnoid (Meningeal) Cyst
- CSF intensity on all pulse sequences
- Primary arachnoid cyst located posteriorly in the spinal canal
- Secondary arachnoid cyst no specific preference
- Lacks vertebral anomalies

(Epi)dermoid Cyst
- Usually in the lumbar spine
- May see sinus tract (20%) or cord tethering

Pathology

General
- Embryology-Anatomy
  - During the third week of embryonic life, the notochord forms and separates the dorsal ectoderm (skin and spinal cord) and the ventral endoderm (foregut)
  - Failure of separation results in a split notochord or a notochord deviated to the left or right of the adhesion
- Etiology-Pathogenesis (spectrum of split notochord syndrome)
  - Dorsal enteric fistula
    - Most severe
    - Connecting the intestinal cavity with the dorsal skin surface, traversing through soft tissues and spine
    - Part(s) of the fistula may obliterate, forming other anomalies
  - Dorsal enteric sinus
    - Blind ending tract with opening on the dorsal skin surface
  - Dorsal enteric enterogenous cyst
    - Prevertebral, intraspinal, postvertebral, mediastinal, or mesenteric in location

- o Dorsal enteric diverticulum
  - ▪ Diverticulum from the dorsal mesenteric border of the bowel
  - o A combination of the above anomalies may be present in one patient
- Epidemiology
  - o Second to fourth decade of life
  - o M: F = 3:2

Microscopic Features
- Thin-walled cyst lined by simple, pseudostratified, or stratified cuboidal or columnar epithelium
- Ciliated epithelium and goblet cells may be present
- Clear or proteinaceous fluid

Clinical Issues
Presentation
- Back pain
- Progressive paraparesis and paresthesia
- Gait disturbance

Natural History
- Progressive neurological deterioration

Treatment
- Surgical excision
- Drainage and partial resection if complete excision not possible

Prognosis
- Significant symptomatic improvement

Selected References
1. Barkovich AJ: Pediatric Neuroimaging. 2nd ed. 510-3, 1995
2. Gao PY et al: Neurenteric cysts: pathology, imaging spectrum, and differential diagnosis. International Journal of Neuroradiology 1:17-27, 1995
3. Geremia GK et al: MR imaging characteristics of a neurenteric cyst. AJNR 9:978-80, 1988

Chiari I, Spine

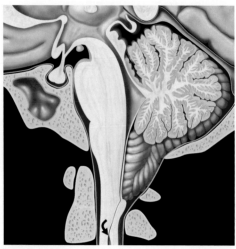

Sagittal midline graphic depicts Chiari I. Note "peg-like", low-lying tonsil with more vertically-oriented sulci. A collapsed syrinx is illustrated (curved arrow). The 4th ventricle is normal.

Key Facts
- Definition: Cerebellar tonsils extending below the foramen magnum
- Classic imaging appearance: Pointed cerebellar tonsils 5 mm below the foramen magnum, with associated syringohydromyelia
- Caused by mild "mismatch" between posterior fossa size (small), cerebellum (normal) ≥ tonsillar "ectopia"
- Tonsils can normally lie below foramen magnum (5 mm or less in adults, slightly more in children < 4y)
- Unless tonsils > 5 mm and/or pointed, probably not Chiari I

Imaging Findings
General Features
- Best imaging clue: Low-lying, pointed (not round), "peg-like" tonsils with vertical (not horizontal) sulci
- 4th occipital sclerotome syndromes (short clivus, craniovertebral segmentation/fusion anomalies) in 50%
CT Findings
- "Crowded" foramen magnum
- Small/absent PF cisterns
- Lateral/3rd ventricle is usually normal
  - +/- Ventriculomegaly
  - Depends upon degree of foramen magnum impaction
MR Findings
- Pointed, triangular-shaped ("peg-like") tonsils
  - ≥ 5 mm below foramen magnum **or**
  - Loss of normal round shape
  - Surrounding CSF effaced
- Small bony PF ≥ low torcular, effaced PF cisterns
- Short clivus ≥ apparent descent 4th ventricle, medulla
  - May be real if LP shunt present
- +/- Syringohydromyelia (14%-75%)

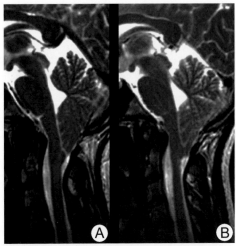

Sagittal T2WIs (A,B) in an asymptomatic patient show findings of classic Chiari I malformation. Note pointed, "peg-like" tonsils 10 mm below foramen magnum. The tonsillar sulci are oriented almost vertically.

Other Modality Findings
- Phase-contrast CSF flow/cord motion MR
  - o Demonstrates pulsatile systolic tonsillar descent
  - o Obstructed CSF flow across foramen magnum

Imaging Recommendations
- MR brain +/- CSF flow studies
- Image the spine to look for
  - o Syrinx, low/tethered cord, or fatty filum

Differential Diagnosis

Acquired Tonsillar Ectopia/Herniation
- Basilar invagination
- "Pull from below": LP/LP shunt ⇒ intracranial hypotension with "sagging" brainstem, acquired tonsillar herniation
- "Push from above"
  - o Chronic VP shunt
    - ▪ Look for thick skull, premature sutural fusion
    - ▪ Arachnoidal adhesions common
  - o Tonsillar herniation 2° ↑ICP, mass effect

Pathology

General
- Genetics
  - o Syndromic/familial
    - ▪ Velocardiofacial/microdeletion chromosome 22
    - ▪ Williams syndrome
    - ▪ Craniosynostosis
- Embryology
  - o Underdeveloped occipital enchondrium ⇒ small posterior fossa vault ⇒ crowded PF ⇒ downward herniated hindbrain ⇒ obstructed

- o Foramen magnum ⇒ lack of communication between cranial/spinal CSF compartments
- Etiology-Pathogenesis-Pathophysiology
  - o Hydrodynamic theory of symptomatic Chiari I
    - Systolic piston-like descent of impacted tonsils/medulla ⇒
    - **Abnormal** pulsatile intraspinal CSF pressure-wave
    - May lead to hydrosyringomyelia
- Epidemiology = 0.01% of population

Gross Pathologic, Surgical Features
- Herniated, sclerotic tonsillar pegs; tonsils grooved by opisthion

Microscopic Features
- Purkinje/granular cell loss

Staging or Grading Criteria
- I = asymptomatic: ≈ 14-50%, treatment controversial
- II = brainstem compression
- III = hydrosyringomyelia

Clinical Issues
Presentation
- Up to 50% asymptomatic
- May mimic multiple sclerosis!
- "Chiari I spells": Cough/headache/ sneeze/syncope
- Symptomatic brainstem compression
  - o Hypersomnolence/central apnea/(infant), sudden death
  - o Bulbar signs (e.g., lower CN palsies)
  - o Neck/back pain, torticollis, ataxia
- Symptomatic syringohydromyelia
  - o Paroxysmal dystonia, unsteady gait, incontinence
  - o Atypical scoliosis (progressive, painful, atypical curve)
  - o Dissociated sensory loss/neuropathy (hand muscle wasting)

Natural History
- Increasing ectopia + ↑ time ⇒ ↑ likelihood symptoms
- Children respond better than adults; treat early

Treatment & Prognosis
- Controversial: Intervention for asymptomatic Chiari I + syrinx
- Direct shunting of symptomatic syrinx obsolete
- Aim = restore normal CSF flow at/around foramen magnum
  - o PF decompression/ resection posterior arch C1
    - >90% ↓ brainstem signs
    - >80% ↓ hydrosyringomyelia
    - Scoliosis arrests (improves in youngest)
  - o +/- Duraplasty, cerebellar tonsil resection
- Anterior decompression/posterior stabilization rarely indicated (some craniocervical anomalies)

Selected References
1. Genitory L et al: Chiari type 1 anomalies in children and adolescents: Minimally invasive management in a series of 53 cases. Childs Nerv Syst 16(10-11): 707-18, 2000
2. Nishikawa M et al: Pathogenesis of Chiari malformations: A morphometric study of the posterior cranial fossa. J Neurosurg 86: 40-7, 1997
3. Menezes AH: Primary craniovertebral anomalies and the hindbrain herniation syndrome (Chiari 1): Data base analysis. Pediatric Neurosurg 23: 260-69, 1995

Myelomeningocele

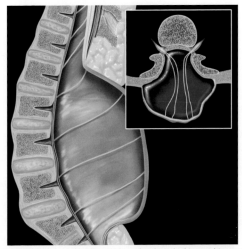

Sagittal drawing depicts a markedly patulous dural sac lacking a skin covering (open dysraphism). Inset shows axial view with wide spinal dysraphism and nerve roots dangling from the ventral placode.

Key Facts
- Synonym(s): Open spinal dysraphism, "spina bifida aperta"
- Definition: Osseous defect of posterior spinal elements that lacks skin covering, permitting exposure of neural tissue, CSF, and meninges to air
- Classic imaging appearance: Wide osseous spinal dysraphism with low-lying cord/roots and post-operative skin closure changes
- Nearly all patients have associated Chiari II malformation
- Rarely imaged prior to skin closure and repair
- Most imaging indications are post-myelomeningocele (MM) closure
  - Complications of surgical repair (tethered cord)
  - Unsuspected associated abnormalities such as diastematomyelia
  - Neurological deterioration from hydrocephalus

Imaging Findings
General Features
- Untreated MM is rarely imaged except with obstetric (fetal) ultrasound
- Best imaging clues: Dilatation of distal canal and thecal sac, low-lying cord, postoperative changes; look also for Chiari II brain findings
CT Findings
- Osseous dysraphism covered with skin; low-lying cord/roots
- Mainly used to detect postoperative complications
  - Spine CT: Diastematomyelia spur, dural constriction, or cord ischemia sequelae (abrupt cord termination)
  - Head CT: Hydrocephalus from VP shunt failure
MR Findings
- Modality of choice for imaging of postoperative complication
  - Wide spinal dysraphism, flared laminae, skin-covered CSF sac
  - Lowlying cord and roots best demonstrated in sagittal plane
    - Low lying cord may not be clinically symptomatic
    - Decision to operate is made on clinical, not radiological grounds

Myelomeningocele

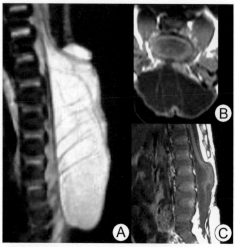

(A,B) Unrepaired myelomeningocele. Sagittal T2WI (A) shows open dysraphism, protruding dural sac. (B) Axial T1WI shows characteristic wide dysraphism, nerve roots dangling from ventral placode. (C) Sagittal T1WI, post-op myelomeningocele (different case), shows typical findings of low-lying cord, distorted nerve roots.

    o Diminished conus pulsation on cine phase contrast CSF flow study

<u>Other Modality Findings</u>
- Obstetric ultrasound: Open neural arch, flared laminae, protruding myelomeningocele sac, and associated Chiari II brain findings ("lemon" sign, "banana" sign, hydrocephalus)

<u>Imaging Recommendations</u>
- Obstetric ultrasound for initial MM diagnosis to assist delivery planning (MM patients are delivered by Caesarian section)
- Head CT for hydrocephalus surveillance
- MR imaging for post-operative spinal imaging indications

Differential Diagnosis
<u>Closed (occult) Spinal Dysraphism</u>
- Also demonstrates dorsal dysraphism; cord may be low-lying
- Distinguished from MM by presence of skin or other cutaneous derivative (e.g. lipoma) covering neural elements

Pathology
<u>General</u>
- General Path Comments
  - o Associations include Chiari II malformation (nearly 100%), syrinx (30-75%), hydrocephalus (80%), diastematomyelia (30 to 45%), callosal dysgenesis, and segmentation anomalies
  - o 10% of MM patients with diastematomyelia have hemimyelocele variation
    - One or both hemicords end in myelomeningocele or other anomaly
- Embryology-Anatomy
  - o All findings result from localized failure of neural tube closure

- The posterior placode surface would normally form the internal ependyma of the neural tube
- The anterior placode surface would normally form the external pia mater cord surface
  - o Lack of closure prohibits separation of neural tissue from cutaneous ectoderm
    - Neural tissue remains attached to skin along lateral placode
    - Relative cord tethering and immobility
    - Mesenchyme cannot migrate inward and is forced to remain anterolateral, preventing the posterior elements from fusing
  - o Dorsal roots arise from anterior placode surface lateral to the ventral roots; both course ventrally through CSF to exit at correct level
- Epidemiology
  - o Incidence 0.6/1000 live births; linked to maternal folate deficiency

Clinical Issues

Presentation

- Typical pre-repair clinical features
  - o Newborn clinically presents with exposed, raw, red, neural tissue placode in the middle of the back
  - o Level of defect is usually lumbosacral (cervical/thoracic level very rare)
    - Level determines severity of neurological deficits
  - o Hydrocephalus secondary to Chiari II malformation
- Typical post-repair clinical features
  - o Fixed neurological deficits, scoliosis, and hydrocephalus
  - o Neurological deterioration suggests a complication
    - Tethered cord, dural ring constriction, cord ischemia, or syringohydromyelia

Treatment

- Myelomeningocele is surgically closed within 48 hours to stabilize neural deficits, prevent infection
  - o Some tertiary centers perform experimental in-utero surgical repair
- Subsequent management is postoperative complications
  - o Untethering of tethered cord
  - o Hydrocephalus management

Prognosis

- Stable postoperative deficit is expected and best outcome possible
- Patients do not improve outcome following repair
- Hydrocephalus and tethered cord determine prognosis for deterioration

Selected References
1. Bowman RM et al: Spina bifida outcome: a 25-year prospective. Pediatr neurosurg 34(3): 114-20, 2001
2. Shurtleff DB et al: Epidemiology of tethered cord with meningomyelocele. Eur J Pediatr Surg 7 suppl 1: 7-11, 1997
3. Barkovich A: Pediatric Neuroimaging. 2nd ed. Philadelphia: Lippincott-Raven, 1996

Dermal Sinus

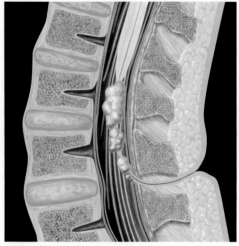

Sagittal illustration of the lumbar spine depicts a dorsal dermal sinus tract extending from the skin surface into the spinal canal. Pearly white epidermoid tumors are present in the cauda equina.

Key Facts
- Synonym: Dorsal dermal sinus
- Definition: Midline epithelial-lined tract extending inward from the skin surface for a variable distance
- Classic imaging appearance
  - Subcutaneous tract between the skin surface and the spine with associated spina bifida
- Other key facts
  - Most common in the lumbosacral (60%) and the occipital (25%) regions
  - Intraspinal extension of the sinus tract occurs in one-half to two-thirds of the cases
  - Associated with dermoid and epidermoid in 30% to 50% of the cases
  - 20% of spinal (epi)dermoids are associated with dermal sinuses
  - Spina bifida frequently present
  - Cord often tethered
  - Meningitis or intraspinal abscess may be the initial presentation
  - CT myelography can supplement MR in evaluating the intraspinal portion of the sinus tract and extramedullary CSF-isointense masses
  - Ultrasound can supplement MR in infants less than one year of age

Imaging Findings
General Features
- Best imaging clue: Hypointense tract in the hyperintense subcutaneous fat deep to the skin surface on T1WI

CT Myelogram Findings
- Spina bifida
- Groove in the lamina or spinous process at the involved level
- Dorsal tenting of the dura
- Intra- or extramedullary (epi)dermoid

Dermal Sinus

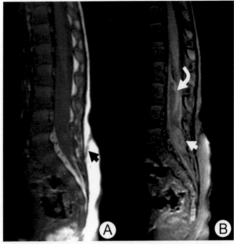

Sagittal T1 pre- (A) and post-gadolinium (B) MR images reveal a subcutaneous hypointense tract (black arrow). There is a mildly enhancing intraspinal mass in the lower lumbar canal (white arrow), with a peripherally enhancing collection more cranially (curved arrow). Dermoid with intradural abscess found at surgery.

MR Findings
- Dermoids may be iso- or hyperintense to cerebral spinal fluid on T1WI
- Epidermoids isointense to cerebral spinal fluid
  - Extramedullary lesion can be very subtle, but may be suggested by nerve root or cord displacement
- Intra- or extramedullary abscess
- Chemical arachnoiditis from ruptured dermoid cyst
- Abscess and arachnoiditis best seen with gadolinium
- Tethered cord

Imaging Recommendations
- Window and level of the MR image may need to be adjusted to delineate the subcutaneous tract
- Heavily T1 weighted sequence (inversion recovery or SPGR) may distinguish extramedullary masses from CSF

Differential Diagnosis
Intraspinal Neoplasm
- No spina bifida or cord tethering
- Diffuse enhancement

Pathology
General
- Embryology-Anatomy
  - The neural tube forms by the infolding and closure of the neural ectoderm
    - As it separates from the cutaneous ectoderm
    - Occurring in the third and fourth week of the embryonic life
    - In a process known as neurulation and disjunction

Dermal Sinus

- Etiology-Pathogenesis
  - Dermal sinus results as focal incorporation of the cutaneous ectoderm into the neural ectoderm during disjunction
  - Bacterial meningitis from retrograde passage of pathogens through the sinus tract
- Epidemiology
  - Early childhood, up to the third decade
  - M: F = 1:1

Gross Pathologic-Surgical Features
- Sinus tract may terminate in
  - Conus medullaris
  - Filum terminale
  - Nerve root
  - Dermoid or epidermoid
- Discrete pearly white tumors
- May see cheesy, oily material in dermoids

Microscopic Features
- Desquamated epithelium in epidermoid
- Skin adnexa in the dermoid

Clinical Issues

Presentation
- Midline sacral dimple or ostium
- Associated hyperpigmented patch, hairy nevus, capillary angioma, or skin tag
- Palpable subcutaneous tract
- Meningitis
- Neurological deficits from mass effect on the spinal cord or cauda equina

Natural History
- Progressive neurological deterioration from cord tethering or as (epi)dermoids enlarge

Treatment
- Surgical excision of the sinus tract and drainage of abscess
- Release of tethered cord
- Long-term antibiotics for infection

Prognosis
- Early surgical intervention usually leads to normal neurological development

Selected References
1. Chen CY et al: Dermoid cyst with dermal sinus tract complicated with spinal subdural abscess. Pediatr Neurol. 2:157-60, 1999
2. Kanev PM et al: Dermoids and dermal sinus tracts of the spine. Neurosurg Clin N Am. 2:359-66, 1995
3. Barkovich AJ et al: MR evaluation of spinal dermal sinus tracts in children. AJNR 12:123-9, 1990

Diastematomyelia

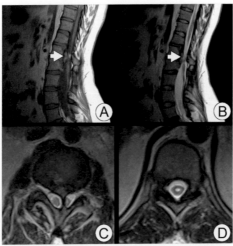

(A,B) Midline sagittal T1WI and T2WI demonstrate a marrow-filled osseous spur at L1 (arrows). Note low-lying conus. (C) Axial T2WI demonstrates the sagittally-oriented osseous spur splitting the spinal cord into two hemicords. (D) Axial T2WI centered above spur shows a single spinal cord with syrinx.

Key Facts
- Synonym(s): Split cord
- Definition: Sagittal division of the spinal cord into two hemicords, each containing a central canal, one dorsal horn, and one ventral horn
- Classic imaging appearance: Two hemicords split in the sagittal plane by a fibrous or osseous spur
- Part of "Split Notochord Syndrome" spectrum
- Associated with other congenital spinal deformities
  - Up to 15–20% of Chiari II malformation patients
  - Vertebral body segmentation anomalies
  - Spinal dysraphism
  - Tethered spinal cord

Imaging Findings
General Features
- Majority occur in lumbar spine (85% between T9-S1)
- Hemicords reunite above and below cleft in most cases
- Spur may be fibrous, osteocartilaginous, or osseous
- +/- hydromyelia
- Frequently see thickening of filum and cord tethering
- Best imaging clue: Split cord and spur is often found at level demonstrating intersegmental fusion
CT Findings
- Two hemicords
- Osseous vertebral segmentation anomalies
- +/- osseous spur (fibrous spurs are usually occult on CT)
MR Findings
- Two hemicords; may see syrinx or hydromyelia
- T1WI - Spur will be isointense if fibrous, and hyperintense if osseous (contains marrow)

Diastematomyelia

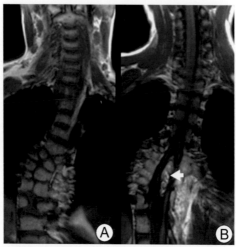

(A) Coronal T1WI shows multiple vertebral body segmentation anomalies with butterfly and hemi-vertebra in conjunction with scoliosis. (B) Spinal cord splits into two hemicords around osseous spur (arrow).

- T2WI – hemicords easy to identify surrounded by bright CSF; best sequence to distinguish presence of one or two dural sacs

Imaging Recommendations
- Begin investigation with MR imaging
  - o T1 and T2 coronal and axial images demonstrate hemicords
  - o Axial T2 weighted images optimally demonstrate composition/location of spur, and presence or absence of syrinx
- Supplement with CT to optimally define spur anatomy if surgical intervention is planned

Differential Diagnosis
Duplicated Spinal Cord (Diplomyelia)
- Often talked about, but exceedingly rare

Pathology
General
- General Path Comments
  - o Strongly associated with other spinal anomalies
  - o Cleft almost always completely splits the cord, with a single cord above and below split
  - o 50% of patients share a dural sac; other 50% demonstrate separate dural tubes
- Etiology-Pathogenesis
  - o Notochord splits but maintains a persistent connection between the gut and dorsal ectoderm
    - ▪ Congenital splitting of the notochord produces a spectrum of "split notochord syndromes"
    - ▪ Degree of abnormality determines which anomalies occur
  - o Notochord directly influences vertebral body formation, thus almost always see vertebral segmentation anomalies

Diastematomyelia

- Epidemiology
  - Uncommon; variable age of symptom onset
  - 5% of congenital scoliosis
  - Females > Males

Gross Pathologic-Surgical Features
- Spinal column nearly always abnormal
  - Segmentation anomalies
  - Spinal dysraphism
  - Tethered cord

Clinical Issues

Presentation
- Nonspecific neurologic symptoms
  - Indistinguishable clinically from tethered cord
- Cutaneous stigmata > 50% of cases
- Orthopedic foot problems = 50% (especially clubfoot)
- Urologic dysfunction

Treatment
- Surgical release of tethered cord and resection of spur

Prognosis
- Stable or progressive disability if untreated
- Up to 90% of patients stabilize or improve following surgery

Selected References
1. Barkovich A: Pediatric neuroimaging. Philadelphia: Lippincott-Raven, 2nd ed, 1996
2. Pang D et al: Split cord malformation: Part I: A unified theory of embryogenesis for double spinal cord malformations. Neurosurgery 31(3): 451-80, 1992
3. Hilal SK et al: Diastematomyelia in children. Radiographic study of 34 cases. Radiology 112(3): 609-21, 1974

Caudal Regression Syndrome

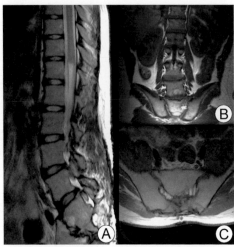

CRS - Group 1. (A) Sagittal T2WI shows "wedge-shaped" distal cord and abnormal cauda equina. Coronal (B) and axial (C) T1WI demonstrate hypoplastic sacrum and pelvis.

Key Facts
- Synonym(s): CRS, sacral agenesis, lumbosacral dysgenesis
- Definition: Constellation of caudal developmental growth abnormalities with associated regional soft-tissue anomalies
- Classic imaging appearance: Lumbosacral dysgenesis with abnormal distal spinal cord
- Other key facts
  - Spectrum of imaging findings ranging in severity from absent coccyx to lumbosacral agenesis
  - 15-20% are infants of diabetic mothers
  - Two main subgroups with distinctive imaging appearances
    - Group 1: More severe caudal dysgenesis with high-lying, club-shaped cord terminus
    - Group 2: Less severe dysgenesis with low-lying, tapered, distal cord tethered by tight filum, lipoma, lipomyelomeningocele, or terminal myelocystocele

Imaging Findings
General Features
- Best imaging clue: Lumbosacral vertebral dysgenesis with abnormal distal spinal cord
CT Findings
- Lumbosacral osseous hypogenesis
- CT depicts soft-tissue anomalies less well than MR imaging
MR Findings
- Vertebral body dysgenesis/hypogenesis
- Hypoplasia of distal spinal cord with distinct "wedge-shaped" cord termination in more severe (Group 1) cases
- Tapered, low-lying, distal cord elongation and tethering in less severe cases (Group 2)

Caudal Regression Syndrome

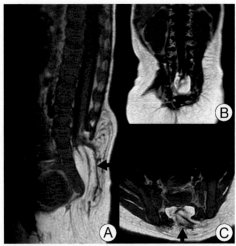

CRS - Group 2. (A) Sagittal T1WI shows mild sacral dysgenesis with abnormal low-lying tapered spinal cord terminating in a large lipoma (arrow). (B) Coronal T1WI shows abnormal cord morphology with sacral dysgenesis. (C) Axial T1WI confirms posterior dysraphism and lipoma (arrow).

   o Look for explanatory anatomical abnormality for tethering

Other Modality Findings
- Plain films document extent of osseous deficiency but not soft tissue abnormalities
- CT or ultrasound abdominal, thoracic, and extremity imaging best characterizes associated tracheo-esophageal fistula, anorectal atresia, renal anomalies, and limb deformities

Imaging Recommendations
- Sagittal T1 and T2 MR imaging to demonstrate extent of lumbosacral deficiency, distal spinal cord morphology, and presence or absence of tethering
- Axial T1 and T2 imaging to delineate extent of osseous spinal narrowing for surgical planning
- CT or ultrasound most helpful to elucidate extent of associated soft tissue anomalies

Differential Diagnosis

Tethered Spinal Cord
- Difficult to discern clinically from mild sacral dysgenesis
- Associated imaging abnormalities help distinguish the two

Closed Spinal Dysraphism
- Posterior dysraphism without severe vertebral column agenesis

Pathology

General
- General Path Comments
  - o Spectrum of severity
  - o Lower extremity deformities, lumbosacral agenesis, anorectal abnormalities, renal/pulmonary hypoplasia characteristic

- Most severe cases demonstrate sirenomelia (lower extremity fusion like a mermaid)
- 20% have associated subcutaneous lesions causing tethering (Group 2 patients)
- Etiology-Pathogenesis
  - Developmental abnormalities within the caudal cell mass before the fourth gestational week
  - Infectious, toxic, or ischemic insults are postulated as initiating subsequent lack of spinal cord and column formation
- Epidemiology
  - Sporadic or syndromic (VACTERL, OEIS, Currarino triad)
  - Nearly all cases sporadic
  - 1/7500 births
  - Male = Female
  - Milder forms > severe forms
  - Affects 1% of offspring from diabetic mothers

Gross Pathologic-Surgical Features
- Degree of vertebral dysgenesis, presence or absence of tethering, and diameter of osseous canal are important factors for surgical planning

Clinical Issues
Presentation
- Broad spectrum ranging from mild foot disorders to complete sensorimotor lower extremity paralysis
  - Flattened buttocks, narrow hips, distal leg atrophy, and talipes deformities
  - Motor level usually higher than sensory level
  - Level of vertebral aplasia correlates with motor but not sensory level
  - Sacral sensory sparing common even in severe cases
- Neurogenic bladder common
- Anorectal anomalies and renal/pulmonary hypoplasia in more severely affected patients

Treatment
- Surgical untethering if clinically symptomatic
- Orthopedic procedures to improve lower extremity functionality
- Addressing associated soft-tissue anomalies

Prognosis
- Variable depending on severity

Selected References
1. Tortori-Donati P et al: Spinal dysraphism: a review of neuroradiological features with embryological correlations and proposal for a new classification. Neuroradiology 42(7): 471-91, 2000
2. Barkovich A: Pediatric neuroimaging. 2nd ed. Philadepphia: Lippincott-Raven, 1996
3. Pang D: Sacral agenesis and caudal spinal cord malformations. Neurosurgery 32(5): 755-78, discussion 778-9, 1993

Segmentation Anomalies

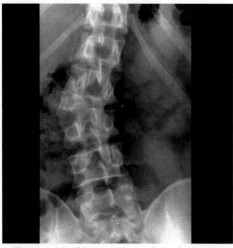

Hemivertebra. There is a right L2 hemivertebra producing focal convex right scoliosis. Tiny rudimentary ribs are noted at T12.

Key Facts
- Definition: Vertebral column malformations due to deranged embryological development
- Classic imaging appearance: Scoliotic patient with deformed vertebral bodies
- May be isolated or syndromal, singular or multiple
  - Association with dysraphism
  - Association with split notochord syndromes
- Term is used to describe several vertebral anomalies
  - Partial or complete failure of formation
    - Vertebral aplasia
    - Hemivertebra
    - Butterfly vertebra
  - Partial duplication
    - Supernumerary hemivertebra
  - Segmentation failure
    - Block vertebra
    - Posterior element dysraphism/fusion (pediculate bar, neural arch fusion)

Imaging Findings
General Features
- Best imaging clue: Look for scoliosis (particularly sharply angulated, single curve, or focal)

CT Findings
- CT best depicts osseous structure
  - Posterior element abnormalities readily identified in axial plane
  - Vertebral body deformity more difficult to evaluate in axial plane

MR Findings
- Most vertebral anomalies seen well in coronal, sagittal planes
- Shows associated abnormalities better than CT

19

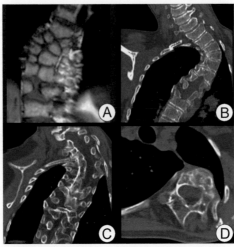

(A) Coronal T1WI shows multiple hemi- and butterfly vertebra with congenital scoliosis. (B) Coronal CT reformat shows segmentation failure producing scoliosis. (C) Multisegment fusion of the right posterior elements. (D) Axial CT demonstrates right pedicular hypoplasia.

- o Diastematomyelia, syrinx
- o Congenital tumor, visceral organ anomalies

Other Modality Findings
- Plain films demonstrate osseous abnormalities well
  - o May be obtained erect to assess weightbearing effect on scoliosis

Imaging Recommendations
- Plain films to evaluate degree of scoliosis with weight bearing
- Multiplanar T1–weighted MR imaging to evaluate vertebral anatomy
- T2WI to evaluate associated cord pathology, compression

Differential Diagnosis

Fracture
- Look for soft-tissue edema, cord injury, appropriate clinical history
- Edges of fracture fragments are noncorticated and irregular

Juvenile Chronic Arthritis
- Difficult to distinguish from cervical block vertebra
- Search for other affected joints, appropriate history

Pathology

General
- General Path Comments
  - o Segmentation anomalies result from disordered vertebral column formation
  - o Thoracolumbar region affected most often
  - o Mildest and most common form is indeterminate (transitional) vertebrae at thoracolumbar, lumbosacral transition
- Embryology-Anatomy
  - o Normal vertebral formation occurs over three sequential periods
  - o Membrane development

- Segmental formation of medial sclerotome (vertebral bodies) and lateral myotome (paraspinal muscles)
  - o Chondrification
    - Sclerotomes separate transversely and join with adjacent sclerotomal halves to form nascent vertebral bodies
    - Paired chondrification sites develop on each side of midline in the vertebral bodies and neural arches
  - o Ossification
    - Chondral skeleton ossifies from single ossification center
- Etiology-Pathogenesis
  - o Total aplasia – failure of both chondral centers to develop
  - o Lateral hemivertebra
    - One chondral center does not develop; ossification center subsequently fails to develop on that side
    - May be supernumerary or replace normal vertebral body
  - o Posterior hemivertebra – later failure at ossification stage
  - o Sagittal cleft ("butterfly") vertebra
    - Separate ossification centers form (but fail to unite) in each paired paramedian chondrification centers
  - o Coronal cleft vertebra – formation and persistence of separate ventral and dorsal ossification centers
  - o Block vertebra – failure of two or more vertebral somites to segment
    - Single or multiple, focal or extensive
    - Lumbar > cervical > thoracic
    - Disc space frequently rudimentary or absent
    - Combined vertebrae may be normal height, short, or tall
    - Frequent association with hemivertebra/absent vertebra above or below the block level, posterior element mal-segmentation
  - o Posterior neural arch anomalies
    - Failure to unite in the midline produces dysraphism (with or without unilateral pedicle aplasia/hypoplasia)
    - Unfused spinous processes most common (in descending frequency) at L5 and S1, C1, C7, T1, and lower thoracic spine
    - Multiple level posterior fusion produces congenital vertebral bars

Clinical Issues
Presentation
- May be asymptomatic or produce abnormal spine curvature
- Neuromuscular scoliosis, neural deficits, limb or visceral defects
  - o Scoliosis usually progressive
- Rarely respiratory failure (impeded chest movement)
Treatment
- Conservative in mild cases
- Surgical fusion to arrest/reverse kyphoscolioisis

Selected References
1. Suh SW et al: Evaluating Congenital spine deformities for intraspinal anomalies with magnetic resonance imaging. J Pediatr Orthop 21(4): 525-31, 2001
2. Jaskwhich D et al: Congenital scoliosis. Curr Opin Pediatr 12(1): 61-6, 2000
3. McMaster MJ et al: Natural history of congenital kyphosis and kyphoscoliosis. A study of one hundred and twelve patients. J Bone Joint Surg Am 81(10): 1367-83, 1999

Craniovertebral Junction

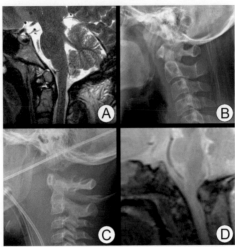

(A) Sagittal T2WI of os odontoideum. (B) Lateral plain film shows congenital hypoplastic dens with normal C1/2 alignment. (C) Atlanto-occipital dislocation with marked distraction of C0/1 facets and malalignment of clivus with dens. (D) Sagittal T2WI reveals severe CVJ stenosis in pediatric Achondroplastic dwarf.

Key Facts
- Synonym(s): CVJ, craniocervical junction
- Definition: Articulation of skull base with cervical spine
- Classic imaging appearance: Variable; reflects underlying pathology
- Abnormalities at this location categorized by etiology
  - Congenital
    - Klippel-Feil, other segmentation disorders
    - Mucopolysaccharidoses
    - Achondroplasia
  - Inflammatory arthritides
    - Rheumatoid arthritis
    - Seronegative spondyloarthropathies
  - Infection
  - Neoplasm
    - Chordoma
    - Chondrosarcoma
    - Metastasis
  - Degenerative arthritis (osteoarthritis)
  - Trauma

Imaging Findings
General Features
- Best imaging clue: Misalignment or malformation of clivus, anterior C1 ring, and/or dens
- Klippel-Feil
  - Fusion starts at C0/1, C1/2, or C2/3 in most cases
  - Fusion may be partial or complete, and affect the vertebral bodies, pedicles, laminae, or spinous processes
- Inflammatory and degenerative arthritides usually manifest fusion or displacement of C1 anterior ring from dens

Craniovertebral Junction

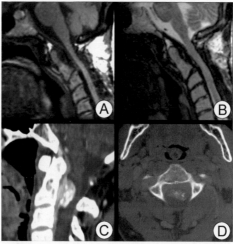

(A,B) Sagittal T1WI, T2WI show marked ligamentous thickening and CVJ stenosis in mucopolysaccharidosis (Hurler's syndrome) patient. (C, D) Sagittal and axial CT images demonstrate calcified enhancing dural-based mass (meningioma) narrowing the ventral C2 canal.

- Tumors, infection show destructive osseous changes and enhance
  - May also show specific imaging characteristics (e.g. chondroid matrix in chondrosarcoma)
- Trauma demonstrates fracture and/or ligamentous abnormality

CT Findings
- Axial images demonstrate bone mineralization, facet status, and canal diameter
- Sagittal and coronal reformations best show alignment and presence/ degree of cranial settling

MR Findings
- Depict soft-tissue structures best
  - Ligamentous disruption, mass lesion, pannus, spinal cord abnormality

Other Modality Findings
- Plain films
  - Show C1/2 articulation well, but are limited for evaluating C0/1
  - Useful for hardware follow-up

Imaging Recommendation
- Axial CT with multiplanar reformations for evaluating osseous structures
- Sagittal and axial T1WI and T2WI to evaluate cord, soft tissues

Differential Diagnosis
- None

Pathology
General
- Congenital CVJ abnormalities are relatively common
  - Klippel-Feil syndrome

- o Os odontoideum
  - Well-defined ossicle at dens tip with anterior C1 arch hypertrophy
  - Not always possible to differentiate from chronic fracture nonunion
- o C1 ring assimilation ("occipitalization") into skull base
  - May be fibrous
  - Many also have C2/3 fusion
- o Dens agenesis (rare)
- Additionally, many acquired disease processes affect CVJ
  - o Inflammatory arthritides (RA, ankylosing spondylitis, psoriatic, Reiter's)
  - o Tumors (chordoma, metastases)
  - o Degenerative arthritis
  - o Trauma
- Etiology-Pathogenesis
  - o Variable – dependent on associated disease process
- Epidemiology
  - o Klippel-Feil syndrome
    - 1/233 to 1/42,000 births
    - Sporadic and familial cases reported; M=F
  - o RA
    - Young to middle age; female to male 3:1
    - Cervical spine involved in 50%; thoracic and lumbar spine rare
    - 33% exhibit C1/2 instability on flexion
  - o Trauma
    - CVJ relatively uncommon site for spine fractures
    - Conversely, CVJ injuries associated with high morbidity/mortality
  - o Osteoarthritis
    - C1/2 degenerative pannus common – rarely causes cord compression

Gross Pathologic-Surgical Features
- Variable – dependant on associated disease process

Clinical Issues
Presentation
- Klippel-Feil - short neck, low posterior hairline, limited cervical motion
  - o Associated abnormalities include Sprengel's deformity, cervical ribs, webbed neck, hemi-vertebrae, spina bifida, visceral anomalies
- Inflammatory arthritis – cord compression, pain, extremity deformity
- Tumor – pain, cranial nerve deficits
- Osteoarthritis – Asymptomatic or painful; typical extremity findings
- Trauma – appropriate history, clinical findings
Treatment
- Correction or amelioration of underlying disease process
- Surgical fusion or decompression
Prognosis
- Variable – dependant on primary disease process

Selected References
1. Smoker WR: MR imaging of the craniovertebral junction. Magn Reson Imaging Clin N Am 8(3): 635-50, 2000
2. Kim FM: Developmental anomalies of the craniocervical junction and cervical spine. Magn Reson Imaging Clin N Am 8(3): 651-74, 2000
3. Menezes AH: Craniovertebral junction anomalies: diagnosis and management. Semin Pediatr Neurol, 4(3): 209-23, 1997

Congenital Spinal Stenosis

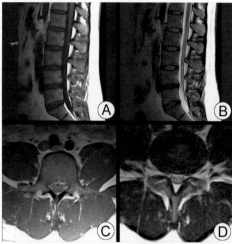

Lumbar short pedicles. (A, B) Sagittal T1WI and T2WI show narrowing of distal canal AP diameter. (C) Axial proton density image confirms that pedicles are short, thick, and more laterally oriented than usual. (D) Axial T2WI reveals L4-5 disc bulge aggravating the congenital spinal stenosis.

Key Facts
- Synonym(s): "Short pedicle" syndrome, congenital short pedicles
- Definition: Reduced AP canal diameter due to short pedicles
- Classic imaging appearance: Short, thickened pedicles, trefoil-shaped lateral recesses, and laterally directed laminae producing central canal AP narrowing; narrowed angle of laminae-best seen on coronal views
- Onset of symptomatic cervical or lumbar stenosis at a younger age than typical of degenerative stenosis
  - Often combined with acquired (degenerative) stenosis
  - Minor acquired abnormalities (bulge, herniation, osteophyte) may cause severe neurologic symptoms

Imaging Findings
General Features
- Best imaging clue: Short, thick pedicles, narrowed AP canal diameter

CT Findings
- Short, thick pedicles, trefoil-shaped lateral recesses, and laterally directed laminae – junction narrowed on coronal reformations
- Reduced AP canal diameter

MR Findings
- Same as CT

Imaging Recommendations
- Sagittal images demonstrate AP canal narrowing, assess for cord compression
- Axial images confirm pedicle configuration and assess severity of canal narrowing

Congenital Spinal Stenosis

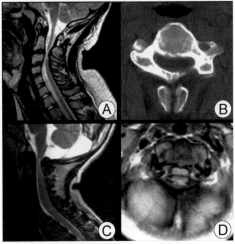

Congenital cervical stenosis. Sagittal T2WI (A) (17M) shows severe cord compression. Axial CT (B) image confirms short, thick pedicles. Inherited cervical stenosis (Morquio's syndrome). Sagittal T2WI (C) shows extensive C1-2 pannus producing severe stenosis. Axial T1WI (D) confirms short AP diameter.

Differential Diagnosis

Acquired Spinal Stenosis
• Assess for subluxation, spondylolysis, degenerative disc/facet changes

Inherited Spinal Stenosis
• Achondroplasia, mucopolysaccharidoses (Morquio syndrome)
• Genetic component
• Often associated with brain, visceral, and/or extremity abnormalities

Pathology

General
• General Path Comments
  ○ Short, thickened pedicles are composed of histologically normal bone
• Epidemiology
  ○ Prevalence in general population difficult to establish
  ○ One study documented congenital cervical stenosis in 7.6% of 262 high school and college football players

Staging or Grading Criteria
• Cervical spine developmental stenosis
  ○ Torg ratio (AP canal diameter/AP vertebral body diameter) < 0.8
  ○ Absolute diameter < 14 mm
    ▪ Must take body habitus into account when measuring
    ▪ Relative dimensions more important than absolute measurement
  ○ Lateral X-ray normally shows articular pillar ending before spinal laminal line
    ▪ If articular pillar takes up entire AP canal dimension on lateral x-ray, canal stenosis is present
• Lumbar spine developmental stenosis
  ○ Absolute AP diameter < 15 mm
  ○ Body habitus influences significance of measurement

Congenital Spinal Stenosis

Clinical Issues

Presentation
- Spinal stenosis symptoms at a younger than expected age
  - Lumbar stenosis presents with usual spinal stenosis symptoms
  - Cervical stenosis patients may present with myelopathy or reversible neurologic deficits ("stingers")
- Cervical cord injury following contact injury in adult athletes

Treatment
- Decompressive laminectomy or laminoplasty

Prognosis
- May be an incidental finding
- Many patients eventually develop symptomatic spinal stenosis

Selected References
1. Boockvar JA et al: Cervical spinal stenosis and sports-related cervical cord neurapraxia in children. Spine 26(24): 2709-13, 2001
2. Smith MG et al: The prevalence of congenital cervical spinal stenosis in 262 college and high school football players. J Ky Med Assoc 91(7): 273-5, 1993
3. Moss A G et al: Computed tomography of the body. Vol two, Philadelphia: W.B.Saunders Company 496-500, 1992

Scoliosis

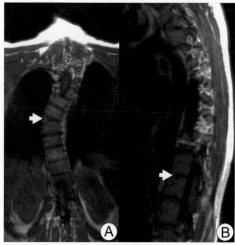

Coronal T1WI of the thoracic spine (A) demonstrates a hemivertebra (arrow) in the mid thoracic spine, resulting in congenital dextroscoliosis. Sagittal T1WI (B) also reveals partial vertebral fusion (arrow).

Key Facts
- Definition: Presence of lateral curvature(s) in the spine, often associated with vertebral rotation
- Classic imaging appearance: S-shaped curvature of the spine
- Idiopathic
  - Most common, 85% of all scoliosis
  - Strongly familial (80%), female predilection (7 to 9:1)
    - Infantile: <3 years of age
    - Juvenile: 4 to 9 years
    - Adolescent: >10 years; most common
- Congenital
  - Result of vertebral anomalies
  - Associated with spinal dysraphic, genitourinary, or cardiac anomalies
- Neuromuscular: Cerebral palsy, poliomyelitis, muscular dystrophy, syringohydromyelia, cord neoplasm
- Posttraumatic or inflammatory: Juvenile rheumatoid arthritis, tuberculosis, radiation therapy
- Dysplasias: Neurofibromatosis, Marfan syndrome, Ehlers-Danlos syndrome
- Neoplasm: Osteoid osteoma
- Imaging evaluation depends on the cause of scoliosis
  - Initial erect anteroposterior and lateral films
  - Posteroanterior projection on follow-up to decrease breast dose
  - Left wrist/hand bone age film
    - Iliac crests on the scoliosis study also provide clue to skeletal maturation
  - Lateral bending films to assess the degree of mobility
  - Cobb method of measuring scoliosis angle

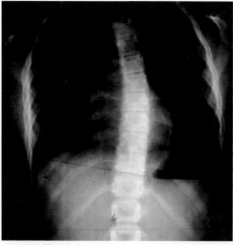

Posteroanterior plain film of the spine in another patient shows mild idiopathic levoscoliosis of the thoracic spine.

- Perpendiculars to a line along the upper endplate of the upper vertebral body of the curve and a line along the lower endplate of the lower vertebral body of the curve
- Same vertebral bodies for follow-up measurements
  o Indications for MRI
    - Congenital scoliosis
    - Juvenile onset: 4 to 9 years
    - Convex left thoracic or thoracolumbar curve
    - Rapid progression of the curve (>1 degree per month)
    - Pain, headache, or neurological signs (cutaneous abdominal reflex) and symptoms (weakness, paresthesia, ataxia)

Imaging Findings

General Features
- Best imaging clue: Lateral curvature(s) in the spine

Plain Film Findings
- Idiopathic
  o Prevalence of typical curvature
    - Convex right thoracic curve> right thoracic and left lumbar> right thoracolumbar> right lumbar
  o Atypical curves
    - Convex left thoracic curve
    - Left thoracolumbar
    - Left cervical
    - Left cervicothoracic
  o Vertebral rotation
  o L5 spondylosis may be present
- Congenital
  o Failure of vertebral formation (wedge vertebra, hemivertebra) or segmentation (pedicle bar, block vertebra)
- Neuromuscular

o Single long curve
- Neurofibromatosis
  o High thoracic acute curvature with posterior vertebral scalloping and rib anomalies

MR Findings (Idiopathic Scoliosis)
- Syringohydromyelia
- Chiari I anomaly
- Cord neoplasm
- Disc disease

Imaging Recommendations
- Coronal T1WI to evaluate vertebral anomalies

Differential Diagnosis

Various Causes of Scoliosis
- Differentiated by clinical history, plain film findings, and supplemented by MRI

Pathology

General
- General Path Comments
  o Scoliosis represents a developmental anomaly of the spine
- Genetics
  o Autosomal dominant transmittance in idiopathic scoliosis
- Epidemiology
  o 0.2% of the population in the United States

Clinical Issues

Presentation
- Idiopathic scoliosis usually detected during physical exam
- Pain from progressive curvature or degenerative disc and facet disease

Natural History
- Curvature less than 30 degrees will not progress when skeletally matured
- Worsening curvature in 25% of the cases
  o During adolescent growth spurts
  o Curves greater than 40 to 50 degrees after skeletal maturity
  o Cardiopulmonary complications from severe scoliosis

Treatment
- Brace
- Electrical stimulation
- Anterior or posterior fusion with instrumentation in skeletally mature patients with >40 degrees of curvature

Prognosis
- Excellent, with proper follow-up and treatment

Selected References
1.   Maiocco B et al: Adolescent idiopathic scoliosis and the presence of spinal cord abnormalities: Preoperative magnetic resonance imaging analysis. Spine 22:2537-41, 1997
2.   Barnes PD et al: Atypical idiopathic scoliosis: MR imaging evaluation. Radiology 186:247-53, 1993
3.   Nokes SR et al: Childhood scoliosis: MR imaging. Radiology 164:791-7, 1987

Tethered Cord

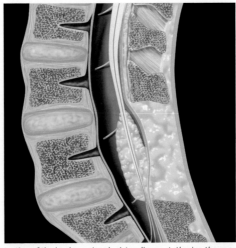

Sagittal illustration of the lumbar spine depicts a lipoma tethering the conus medullaris at L5. The dural sac is mildly widened at this level. In addition, spina bifida is present.

Key Facts
- Definition: Low-lying conus medullaris tethered by a mass, a short and thick filum terminale (tight filum terminale), or scar tissue from prior surgical repair of spinal dysraphism
- Classic imaging appearance: Conus below L2 inferior endplate with associated tethering mass or thick filum
- Other key facts
  - The conus terminates at or above the inferior aspect of L2 in more than 98% of the normal adult population
  - In the remainder 2% or less, the conus reaches the L3 level
  - Clinical tethering may occur with a normal conus level
    - An abnormal filum (fibrolipoma of the filum or a thickened filum) invariably present
  - The normal filum has a diameter less than 2 mm
    - Measured at the L5-1 level
  - Small lipoma in the filum terminale may be an incidental finding
    - Must be correlated clinically for symptoms of tethering
  - MRI is the imaging modality of choice

Imaging Findings
General Features
- Best imaging clue
  - Filum thickened > 2 mm at the L5-1 level on axial MRI
  - Fatty mass associated with the filum
CT Findings
- Scoliosis, spina bifida, vertebral fusion and segmentation anomalies
MR Findings
- Spinal lipomas: Lipomyelo(meningo)cele, intradural lipoma, and fibrolipoma of filum terminale

Tethered Cord

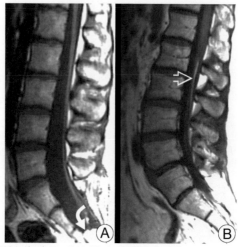

Sagittal T1WI in the first patient (A) demonstrates an elongated cord extending to the S2 segment, tethered by an intraspinal lipoma (curved arrow). In a second patient without any symptoms (B), a fibrolipoma of the filum is present (open arrow), with the conus terminating at the normal location of L1.

- Myelo(meningo)cele
- Diastematomyelia
- Tight filum terminale
  - Conus below the inferior aspect of L2, often tethered by a lipoma
  - Widened dural sac
  - Thickened filum
- Intradural scar tissue from previous surgery
- Dorsal location of the conus medullaris and filum terminale in the thecal sac
- Syringohydromyelia/myelomalacia in the conus or the cord
  - Adjacent to the tethering lesion

Ultrasound Findings
- Useful in children less than one year of age
- Lack of spinal cord pulsation suggestive of cord (re)tethering

Imaging Recommendations
- Phase contrast technique may reveal decreased cervical cord motion in patients with tethering

Differential Diagnosis

Early Post-surgical Low-lying Conus
- Cannot exclude retethering
- Ultrasound to evaluate spinal cord pulsation
- Surgical exploration if retethering is a clinical concern

Low-lying Conus as a Normal Variant
- Normal filum on axial imaging
- No filum lipoma

Tethered Cord

Pathology

General

- General Path Comments
  - o Tethering impairs the oxidative metabolism of the cord and stretches the arterioles and venules
    - ▪ Possibly leading to syringohydromyelia/myelomalacia
- Embryology-Anatomy
  - o The fetal conus "ascends" in the spinal canal
    - ▪ As the most distal portion of the spinal cord undergoes retrogressive differentiation
    - ▪ Vertebral bodies demonstrate relatively rapid growth compared to the remaining cord
- Etiology-Pathogenesis
  - o Spinal lipomas: Lipomyelo(meningo)cele, intradural lipoma, and fibrolipoma of filum terminale
  - o Myelo(meningo)cele
  - o Diastematomyelia
  - o Tight filum terminale
    - ▪ Incomplete retrogressive differentiation
    - ▪ Failure of the fibers of filum terminale to lengthen
  - o Intradural scar tissue from prior surgery
- Epidemiology
  - o Tight filum terminale commonly discovered during growth spurts (childhood or adolescence)
  - o May present in elderly with onset of senescent kyphosis

Clinical Issues

Presentation

- Cutaneous manifestations of lipomyelo(meningo)cele, myelo(meningo)cele, or diastematomyelia
- Low back or leg pain
- Lower extremity stiffness, numbness, weakness, and abnormal reflexes
- Muscular atrophy
- Spastic gait
- Urinary bladder dysfunction
- Scoliosis and foot deformities

Natural History

- Progressive and irreversible neurological impairment

Treatment

- Early prophylactic surgery
- Resect the tethering mass, release the cord, and repair the dura

Prognosis

- Improvement or stabilization of most neurological deficits
- Urinary bladder dysfunction resolves in less than 10% of the cases

Selected References
1. Barkovich AJ: Pediatric Neuroimaging. 2nd ed. 491-6, 1995
2. Raghavan N et al: MR imaging in the tethered spinal cord syndrome. AJR 152:843-52, 1989
3. Hall WA et al: Diagnosis of tethered cords by magnetic resonance imaging. Surg Neurol 30:60-4, 1988

Conjoined Nerve Roots

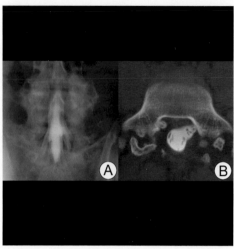

(A) AP post-myelogram plain film shows conjoined roots with aberrant enlarged root sleeve exiting at left S1 foraminal level. (B) Axial CT myelogram image confirms enlarged left S1 root sleeve containing two nerve roots (and incidental spondylolysis).

Key Facts
- Synonym: Composite nerve root sleeve
- Definition: Aberrant root sleeve contains two instead of one nerve root
- Classic imaging appearance: Unilateral enlarged root sleeve containing two roots originating midway between the contralateral positions of two contributing nerve roots
- Occurs throughout spine; most commonly reported in the lumbar spine (L4/5, L5/S1, and L3/4 in order of frequency)
- Important anatomical variant to identify prior to spinal surgery
- Dorsal root ganglia contrast enhancement, enlargement of foraminal neural structures may lead to misdiagnosis as nerve sheath tumor

Imaging Findings
General Features
- Best imaging clue: Enlarged root sleeve contains two roots originating midway between expected dural sac exit of two contributing nerve roots
CT Findings
- Asymmetric anomalous origin of an enlarged nerve root sleeve
- Supernumerary nerve roots on CT myelography
- Possible osseous foraminal enlargement compared to contralateral side
MR Findings
- Asymmetric anomalous origin of an enlarged nerve root sleeve
  - Roots usually exit separately at expected neural foraminal levels
  - Sometimes two roots exit through same (usually lower) foramen
    - In this case will see a CSF-filled foramen without dorsal root ganglion (DRG) at one level and two enhancing DRGs in the other foramen
Other Modality Findings
- Myelography – enlarged aberrant root sleeve leaves dural sac in between contralateral origins of conjoined roots

Conjoined Nerve Roots

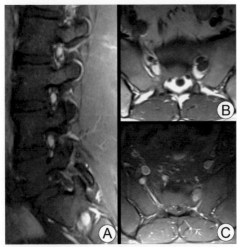

(A) Enhanced fat saturated sagittal T1WI shows normally enhancing DRG at all levels except left L5/S1 foramen. Two enhancing DRGs are seen within the S1 foramen. Axial pre- (B) and post- (C) enhanced T1WI show two DRGs within the left S1 neural foramen.

- o Roots may then separate and exit through appropriate foramina or remain joined and exit through a single foramen

Imaging Recommendations
- Sagittal and axial MR T1WI and T2WI
  - o Sagittal image slice prescription must extend lateral to neural foramen bilaterally
  - o Contrast will show enhancing DRG
- CT myelography excellent for demonstrating relationship of root sleeve to osseous structures

Differential Diagnosis
Nerve Sheath Tumor
- Neurofibroma or Schwannoma mimic
- Contrast enhancement of dorsal root ganglia and enlargement of neural structures within the foramina must not be confused for schwannoma
- Larger tumors show a dumbbell configuration as intradural tumor passes through the dural sleeve into extradural space

Pathology
General
- General Path Comments
  - o More commonly detected at autopsy than on imaging studies
  - o Much more commonly detected in the lumbar spine than cervical or thoracic spine
- Epidemiology
  - o Prevalence of conjoined lumbar nerve roots is generally reported from 0.3 - 2%, but has been reported as high as 10.6%

Gross Pathologic-Surgical Features
- Most commonly unilateral

Conjoined Nerve Roots

- Composite root sleeve generally originates from the dural sac at a point halfway between the expected positions of the two sleeves it replaces, and is bigger than a normal sleeve
  o The two contained nerve roots often leave the spinal canal through separate neural foramina
  o Less commonly the two roots leave the canal through a single foramina (usually that of the lower root)
- Failure to correctly appreciate this anatomical variant may lead to misdiagnosis as nerve root tumor or operation at the wrong level for radiculopathy

Clinical Issues
Presentation
- Generally asymptomatic in and of itself
- May be associated with radiculopathy
Treatment
- Generally none indicated
- Surgical decompression may be indicated in selected patients with documented concordant radiculopathy

Selected References
1. Prestar FJ: Anomalies and malformations of lumbar spinal nerve roots. Minim Invasive Neurosurg 39(4): 133-7, 1996
2. Firooznia H et al: Normal correlative anatomy of the lumbosacral spine and its contents. Neuroimaging clinics of North America 3(3): 411-24, 1993
3. Phillips LH et al: The frequency of intradural conjoined lumbosacral dorsal nerve roots found during selective dorsal rhizotomy. Neurosurgery 33(1): 88-90, discussion 90-1, 1993

Ventriculus Terminalis

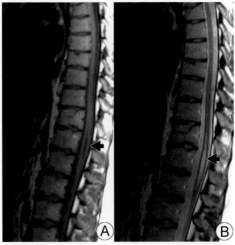

Ventriculus terminalis. (A, B) Sagittal T1WI and T2WI show mild CSF signal intensity dilatation of the distal central canal at the conus level (arrows). No cord signal abnormality, mass, or dilatation of the proximal cord is seen to imply the presence of a syrinx.

Key Facts
- Synonym(s): Terminal ventricle, fifth ventricle
- Definition: Normal slight expansion of the central spinal cord canal at the distal conus and/or proximal filum
- Classic imaging appearance: CSF density/signal intensity within dilated distal central canal
- Typically an incidental finding
- Rarely can become abnormally dilated and symptomatic, necessitating treatment
- Must distinguish from cystic cord neoplasm

Imaging Findings
General Features
- Best imaging clue: Mild cystic dilatation of distal central canal without cord signal abnormality or enhancement
CT Findings
- Mild dilatation of distal central canal
- No associated mass lesion or enhancement
MR Findings
- Slight expansion of the distal central canal
- Contents show CSF signal intensity on ALL sequences
- Conus is at normal level (T12 to L2)
- No cord signal abnormality, mass effect, or enhancement
Other Modality Findings
- Ultrasound – Mild anechoic central dilatation of distal conus
Imaging Recommendations
- Newborns
  o Ultrasound is accurate for screening babies for congenital anomalies

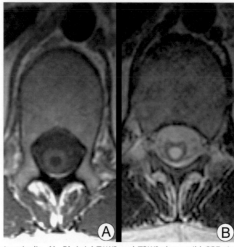

Ventriculus terminalis. (A, B) Axial T1WI and T2WI show mild CSF signal intensity dilatation of the distal central canal at the conus. Despite the degree of central canal dilatation in this asymptomatic patient, there is no cord signal abnormality or suggestion of mass to imply a pathological condition.

- o Can distinguish ventriculus terminalis from syrinx or distal cord neoplasm
- o Abnormal findings should be confirmed with MR imaging
- Children, adults, and infants with positive ultrasound studies
  - o MR imaging with thin section sagittal T1WI and T2WI (3 mm slice thickness) to exclude syrinx
  - o Axial T1WI and T2WI (4 mm slice thickness) from distal cord to sacrum to exclude occult dysraphism or filum thickening
  - o Postcontrast T1WI in both planes to exclude mass

Differential Diagnosis
Hydrosyringomyelia
- Progressive expansion and cephalic extension of ventriculus terminalis
- Cystic expansion of the distal one-third (or more) of the cord
- Isolated finding or associated with congenital spine anomalies
Cystic Neoplasm
- Differentiated by cord signal changes, cord expansion, and contrast enhancement of solid portions
Cystic Myelomalacia
- History of trauma or other cord insult
- Associated cord atrophy

Pathology
General
- General Path Comments
  - o Normal microscopic histology
  - o Longitudinal diameter 8–10 mm, transverse diameter 2–4 mm
  - o Size variable throughout life
    - Smallest in middle age

Ventriculus Terminalis

- Largest in early childhood and old age
- Embryology-Anatomy
  - Positioned between tip of conus medullaris and filum terminale origin
  - Forms during embryogenesis as a result of canalization and retrogressive differentiation of caudal end of developing spinal cord
    - Occurs at the point of union between the central canal portion formed by neurulation and the portion formed by caudal cell mass canalization
  - Usually regresses in size during the first weeks after birth
    - Persistence leads to identification in children or adults
- Epidemiology
  - Can be identified at any age
  - 2.6 % of normal children have a visible ventriculus terminalis cavity
  - Less commonly identified in adults
    - Primarily an autopsy curiosity until advent of MR imaging

Microscopic Features
- Cystic cavity lined by ependymal cells

Clinical Issues

Presentation
- Incidental finding on imaging performed for unrelated indications

Treatment
- No treatment indicated for incidental finding
- Surgical decompression and management of associated abnormalities in the rare cases with symptomatic dilated cysts

Prognosis
- No effect on mortality or morbidity

Selected References
1. Kriss VM et al: Sonographic appearance of the ventriculus terminalis cyst in the neonatal spinal cord. J Ultrasound Med, 19(3): 207-9, 2000
2. Matsubayashi R et al: Cystic dilatation of ventriculus terminalis in adulta: MRI. Neuroradiolgy, 40(1): 45-7, 1998
3. Coleman LT et al: Ventriculus terminalis of the conus medullaris: MR findings in children. AJNR AM J Neuroradiol, 16(7): 1421-6, 1995

Lipomyeloschisis

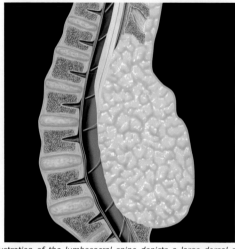

Sagittal illustration of the lumbosacral spine depicts a large dorsal skin-covered lipoma, with an adherent ventral neural placode, contiguous with the subcutaneous fat through a spina bifida defect.

Key Facts
- Synonym: Lipomyelocele/lipomyelomeningocele
- Definition
  - Lipomyelocele is a neural placode-lipoma complex contiguous with subcutaneous fat through a spina bifida
  - Lipomyelomeningocele is a lipomyelocele with a meningocele
- Classic imaging appearance: Subcutaneous fatty mass contiguous with the neural placode/lipoma
- Other key facts
  - 20% to 50% of occult spinal dysraphism
  - Both are covered by skin and fat
  - Cord always tethered
  - Associated vertebral anomalies: Butterfly vertebrae, hemi- vertebrae, fused vertebrae
  - Terminal hydromyelia may be present
  - The lipoma may be asymmetric with rotation of the placode-lipoma complex
  - Most common in the lumbosacral region
  - MRI is the imaging modality of choice for initial evaluation
  - MRI not useful for early postoperative evaluation of re-tethering as the position of the conus is often unchanged immediately after surgery

Imaging Findings
General Features
- Best imaging clue: Spina bifida and overlying fatty mass
CT Findings
- Dorsal spinal dysraphism
- Lucent dorsal lipoma with associated ventral neural placode
- Lipoma contiguous with the subcutaneous fat and tethered cord/placode

Lipomyeloschisis

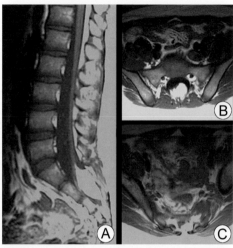

Sagittal T1WI (A) demonstrates a neural placode-lipoma complex in the dorsal sacral canal. Axial T1WI (B) confirms the spina bifida and shows a connection between the lipoma and the subcutaneous fat (C).

Differential Diagnosis

Intradural Lipoma
- Enclosed within an intact overlying dura
- Most commonly in the cervical and thoracic spine
- Lack of cutaneous manifestations

Myelocele/Myelomeningocele
- Not covered by skin or subcutaneous fat
- No lipoma attached to the neural placode

Pathology

General
- Embryology-Anatomy
  - The neural tube forms by the infolding and closure of the neural ectoderm
    - As it separates from the cutaneous ectoderm
    - Occurring in the third and fourth week of the embryonic life
    - In a process known as neurulation and disjunction
- Etiology-Pathogenesis
  - Lipomyeloschisis results from the premature disjunction of the neural ectoderm from the cutaneous ectoderm
  - Mesenchyme is incorporated between the neural folds
  - Neural folds remain open, forming the neural placode at the site of premature disjunction
  - The ependymal lining of the primitive neural tube induces the mesenchyme to form fat
- Epidemiology
  - Female predominance
  - Presents at birth through infancy

Lipomyeloschisis

Clinical Issues
Presentation
- Midline or parasagittal skin covered lumbosacral mass
- Associated skin dimple, tag, hemangioma, or tuft of hair
- Lower extremity paraparesis
- Sacral dermatomal sensory loss
- Bladder and bowel dysfunction
- Foot deformities

Natural History
- Progressive and potentially irreversible neurological impairment from cord tethering or enlarging lipoma

Treatment
- Early prophylactic surgery (less than one year of age) to untether the cord, resect the lipoma, and reconstruct the dura

Prognosis
- Neurologically intact patients at the time of surgery usually remain intact on long-term follow-up
- Bladder dysfunction usually persists if not operated early in infancy
- Symptomatic retethering up to 10% of the cases, occurring weeks to years after the initial surgery

Selected References
1. Barkovich AJ: Pediatric Neuroimaging. 2nd ed. 491-6, 1995
2. Sutton LN: Lipomyelomeningocele. Neurosurgery Clinics of North America 6:325-38, 1995
3. Kaney PM et al: Management and long-term follow-up review of children with lipomyelomeningocele, 1952-1987. J Neurosurg 73:48-52, 1990

Scheuermann's Disease

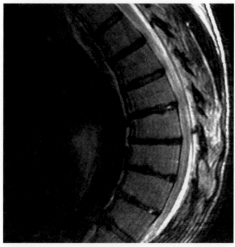

Midline sagittal T2WI demonstrates four consecutive thoracic vertebrae each wedged 5 degrees or more. Disc space narrowing and end-plate irregularities are also present.

Key Facts
- Synonym: Kyphosis dorsalis juvenilis
- Classic imaging appearance
  - Three or more contiguous thoracic vertebrae
  - > or = 5 degrees of anterior wedging
- Other key facts
  - 30% to 50% with associated spondylolysis
  - 75% thoracic involvement
  - 20% to 25% thoracolumbar
  - < 5% lumbar
  - Cervical involvement uncommon
  - Atypical Scheuermann's disease
    - Only one or two vertebral bodies involved
    - No anterior wedging
    - Other findings same as typical Scheuermann's disease

Imaging Findings
General Features
- Best imaging clue: Thoracic kyphosis in a teenage patient
Radiography Findings
- Anterior vertebral body wedging
- Endplate irregularity
- Narrowing of the disc space
- Limbus vertebrae
MR Findings
- In addition to the above
  - Schmorl's node formation
  - Disc extrusions

Scheuermann's Disease

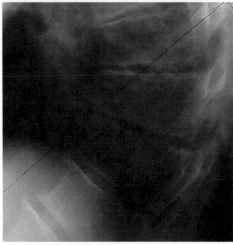

In another patient, sagittal plain film radiography of the thoracic spine demonstrates three consecutive vertebrae each with mild anterior wedging. In addition, there are associated end-plate irregularities.

Differential Diagnosis
<u>Insufficiency Vertebral Compression Fractures</u>
- Underlying osteopenia from various causes
<u>Traumatic Compression Fractures</u>
- Extensive marrow edema

Pathology
<u>General</u>
- Genetics
  - Familial tendency
- Embryology-Anatomy
  - Biochemical abnormality in the matrix of cartilaginous vertebral end plates
    - Diminished number or thickness of collagen fibers
    - Increased proteoglycan content
- Etiology-Pathogenesis
  - Chronic repetitive trauma in a skeletally immature person
    - Weight lifting, gymnastics, and other spine loading sports
    - Hard physical labor
  - Disc extrusions through congenitally weakened regions of vertebral end plates
    - Disc space loss
    - Limbus vertebrae
    - Schmorl's node
  - Delayed growth in the anterior portion of the vertebrae
  - Normal growth in the posterior portion of the vertebrae
- Epidemiology
  - Peak incidence: 13 to 17 years
  - Prevalence: 0.4% to 8%
  - Slight male predominance (2:1 in some reports)

Scheuermann's Disease

Clinical Issues

Presentation

- Principal presenting symptom: Kyphosis
- Thoracic pain and tenderness, worsened by activity
- Generalized fatigue
- Rare myelopathy from kyphosis or from thoracic disc herniations

Natural History

- Develops during the teenage years
- Increases in magnitude during the adolescent growth spurt
- Mild progression after growth is complete
- Severe deformity uncommon

Treatment

- Observation
  - Indications
    - Growth still remains
    - Kyphotic deformity less than 50 degrees
  - Elimination of the specific strenuous activity
  - Analgesics
  - Spine exercises
- Brace treatment
  - Indications
    - At least one year of growth remains
    - < 75 degree kyphosis
    - At least partial correction of the kyphosis on hyperextension
- Surgical treatment
  - Indications
    - > 75 degree kyphosis in a skeletally immature person
    - > 60 degree kyphosis in the mature person
    - Excessive pain
  - Posterior instrumentation and fusion
  - Anterior and posterior fusion

Prognosis

- Brace treatment
  - Effective in preventing kyphosis progression
  - Initial improvement of 20% to 30% in kyphosis one year after treatment
  - Final kyphosis correction up to 50%
- Surgical treatment
  - Posterior surgical approach only may result in loss of the initial correction
  - Combined anterior and posterior approach result in 39% to 59% of correction

Selected References
1. Tala VT et al: Postural kyphosis and Scheuermann's disease. Seminars in Spine Surgery 4:216-24, 1992
2. Blumenthal SL et al: Lumbar Scheuermann's. a clinical series and classification. Spine 12:929-32, 1987
3. Ippolito E et al: Juvenile kyphosis; histological and histochemical studies. J Bone Joint Surg 63: 175-82, 1981

Back Pain in Children

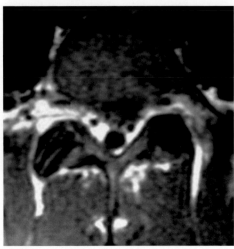

Axial T1WI at L5-S1 in an adolescent demonstrates central and left central disc protrusion, displacing the traversing left S1 nerve root.

Key Facts
- Prepubertal children
  - Back pain a rare functional complaint
  - When present, underlying causes should be sought
- Adolescent children
  - Estimates of low back pain prevalence range between 8% to 50%, increasing with age
  - Annual incidence between 12% to 22%, increasing with age
  - 8% with recurrent or continuous low back pain
  - 2% to 3% with recurrent or continuous low back pain into early adulthood
- Degenerative disc disease
  - Definition: Degenerative changes in the lumbar intervertebral discs
  - Classic imaging appearance: Disc height loss, desiccation, and herniation
  - Correlates with low back pain in adolescence
    - Occurs after growth spurt
    - Increases linearly with age into adulthood
  - 33% of 15 year olds in one series had degenerated discs
    - 89% of those with recurrent low back pain versus 26% of asymptomatic individuals
- Other causes of back pain in children
  - Spondylolysis
    - 5% to 7% asymptomatic prevalence in general population
    - Active athletes may have pars lysis due to stress fracture
  - Spondylolisthesis
  - Spondylodiscitis
  - Scheuermann's disease
  - Neoplasms (osteoid osteoma, leukemia, eosinophilic granuloma)
  - Tethered cord

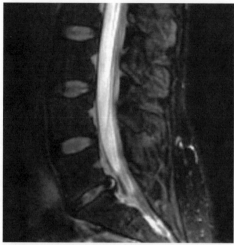

Sagittal T2WI with fat saturation of the lumbar spine in another patient shows an anular tear at L5-S1 with associated disc bulge and mild disc height loss.

- Indications for imaging workup
  - Young age (< 5 years of age)
  - Chronic and recurrent pain
  - Functional disability and limited motion
  - Fever
  - Neurologic signs and symptoms

Imaging Findings: Degenerative Disc Disease
General Features
- Best imaging clue: T2 hypointensity in the intervertebral disc
- Radionuclide study may be useful in cases of spondylolysis, osteoid osteoma, and occult infection

CT Findings
- Disc herniation
- Disc height loss on sagittal reformation
- Endplate irregularities

MR Findings
- Narrowed disc space
- Disc desiccation on T2WI
- Anular tear
- Disc herniation
- Scheuermann's disease-type changes

Differential Diagnosis
Discitis
- Hyperintense disc on T2WI
- Endplate erosive changes
- Subchondral marrow T2 hyperintensity in adjacent vertebral bodies abutting the disc

Back Pain in Children

Pathology
Q <u>General</u>
- Etiology-Pathogenesis
  - o Poorly understood in adolescents with degenerative disc disease

Clinical Issues
<u>Presentation</u>
- Low back pain
<u>Natural History</u>
- Self-limited
- Small percentage with recurrent or continuous symptoms
<u>Treatment</u>
- Conservative
- Bed rest
- Analgesic medications
<u>Prognosis</u>
- Good
- 8% with recurrent or continuous low back pain
- 2% to 3% with symptoms continuing into early adulthood

Selected References
1. Salminen JJ et al: Recurrent low back pain and early disc degeneration in the young. Spine 24:1316-21, 1999
2. Leboeuf-Yde C et al: At what age does low back pain become a common problem? A study of 29,424 individuals aged 12-41 years. Spine 23:228-34, 1998
3. Erkintalo MO et al: Development of degenerative changes in the lumbar intervertebral disk: Results of a prospective MR imaging study in adolescents with and without low-back pain. Radiology 196:529-33, 1995

Dural Dysplasias

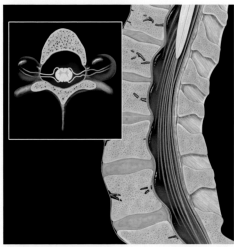

Posterior vertebral body scalloping and patulous dural sac characterize dural ectasia. Inset depicts extensive vertebral body scalloping with lateral meningoceles.

Key Facts
- Synonym: Dural ectasia
- Definition: Expansile dural sac morphology causing remodeling of spinal canal
- Classic imaging appearance: "C" shaped scalloping of the posterior vertebral bodies and patulous thecal sac
- Three disease categories produce posterior vertebral scalloping
  - Dural ectasia
  - Increased intraspinal pressure
  - Congenital vertebral dysplasia
- Recognition of specific imaging clues and integration of available clinical data permits a more specific diagnosis
- Dural dysplasia is most commonly associated with Neurofibromatosis type 1, Marfan's syndrome, Homocystinuria, and Ehler-Danlos syndrome

Imaging Findings
General Features
- Best imaging clue: Smooth scalloping of the posterior vertebral bodies in conjunction with enlarged dural sac

CT Findings
- Smooth remodeling of posterior vertebral body expanding central canal
  - Easiest to appreciate on sagittal reformatted images
- CSF density sac
- May also find imaging stigmata of associated etiological diseases
  - Osteoporosis suggests Homocystinuria
  - Pseudoarthrosis suggests NF-1

MR Findings
- Enlarged CSF space, remodeled posterior vertebral bodies
- Most useful modality to exclude syrinx, tumor, or other soft tissue cause of canal enlargement before finding is ascribed to dural ectasia

Dural Dysplasias

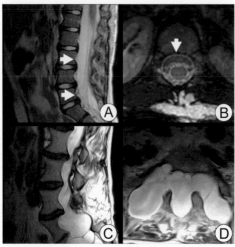

Sagittal T2WI (A), axial FSEIR (B) scans in a patient with NF-1 show smooth posterior vertebral scalloping (arrows). Note hyperintense subcutaneous plexiform neurofibroma on axial image. (C,D) Sagittal and axial T2WIs in a patient with Marfan syndrome show extensive vertebral scalloping, large lateral meningoceles.

Modality Findings
- Plain films show same findings as CT, and may demonstrate pertinent extremity findings that permit a specific diagnosis

Imaging Recommendations
- MR imaging shows osseous abnormalities well; most helpful technique to exclude tumor, syrinx, or other related anatomical abnormalities

Differential Diagnosis

Congenital Vertebral Dysplasias
- Achondroplasia, Mucopolysaccharidoses, osteogenesis inperfecta (tarda)
- Search for appropriate family history and clinical stigmata

Cauda Equina Syndrome of Ankylosing Spondylitis (AS)
- Irregular expansion of lumbar canal
- Caused by dural ectasia thought due to proliferative inflammatory synovium; associated cauda equina symptoms
- Stigmata of AS typically present

Spinal Canal Tumor or Syrinx
- Astrocytoma, ependymoma, idiopathic syrinx
- Characteristic imaging findings will lead to correct diagnosis

Pathology

General
- General Path Comments
  o All congenital dural dysplasias result from genetic predisposition that causes abnormal connective tissue
  o Causative enzymatic deficiency is well defined for each disorder
- Genetics
  o NF-1: Autosomal dominant, gene locus on chromosome 17q12
  o Marfan's: Autosomal dominant

Dural Dysplasias

- o Homocystinuria: Autosomal recessive
- o Ehlers-Danlos: Autosomal dominant
- Epidemiology
  - o NF-1: 1 in 4000; 50% new mutations
  - o Marfan's: No race or gender predominance
  - o Homocystinuria: Autosomal recessive, Northern European ancestry
  - o Ehlers-Danlos: M > F; Caucasian, European descent
- Etiology-Pathogenesis
  - o Marfan's syndrome: Primary connective tissue defect unknown
  - o Ehlers-Danlos: > 10 different types of collagen synthesis defects
  - o Homocystinuria: Cystathionine synthetase deficiency

Gross Pathologic-Surgical Features

- Dural dysplasia is usually incidental
- Morbidity and mortality primarily related to vascular pathology
  - o Fragility and predisposition to arterial dissection or aneurysm

Clinical Issues

Presentation

- Often an incidental finding in patients imaged for associated concerns
- Clinical presentation depends on congenital disease
  - o NF-1: Plexiform neurofibromas, optic nerve gliomas and other astrocytomas, café-au-lait spots, axillary freckling, extremity pseudoarthrosis
  - o Marfan's syndrome: Tall, joint hypermobility, arachnodactyly, kyphoscoliosis, joint and lens dislocations
  - o Homocystinuria: Tall, arachnodactyly, scoliosis, mental retardation, seizures, lens dislocations
  - o Ehlers-Danlos: Tall, thin hyperelastic skin, hypermobile joints, fragile connective tissue

Treatment

- Treatment is directed toward addressing underlying etiology

Prognosis

- Variable depending on etiology

Selected References
1. Villeirs GM et al: Widening of the spinal canal and dural ectasia in Marfan's syndrome: assessment by CT. Neuroradiology, 41(11): 850-4, 1999
2. Fattori R et al: Importance of dural ectasia in phenotypic assessment of Marfan's syndrome. Lancet, 354(9182): 910-3, 1999
3. Raff ML et al: Joint hypermobility syndromes. Curr Opin Rheumatol, 8(5): 459-66, 1996

TRAUMA

Hangman's Fracture

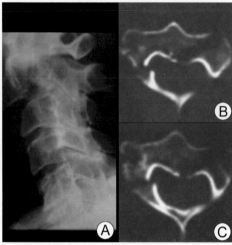

Lateral X-ray (A) demonstrates fractures through pedicles of C2, anterior dislocation of C2 body and C1 relative to C3. Axial CT (B, C) shows fracture of right C2 pedicle, the fracture on the left extends into the body of C2.

Key Facts
- Synonym: Traumatic spondylolisthesis of the axis (TSA)
- Definition: Bilateral avulsion of the C2 body from its arch
- Classic imaging appearance: Bony vertical defects through pedicles of C2 on lateral X-ray, with anterior displacement of C2 vertebral body (Vb) on C3, laminae of C2 and laminal line remaining aligned with laminal line of C3
  - Can see alignment preserved despite fracture
  - Soft-tissue swelling anterior to C2 common
    - CT defines components of fracture to best advantage
    - May see various patterns of arch, Vb disruption

Imaging Findings
General Features
- Best imaging clue: Lateral displacement of articular masses of C1 from those of C2 on open mouth view
CT Findings
- Multiple fractures of C1 arch typical
- Both anterior and posterior arch fractures are seen only in minority
- Posterior arch fractured more often than anterior
- Lateral masses alone may be fractured
- A single site of arch fracture may occur
- Look for avulsion of inner pillar at insertion of transverse ligament
MR Findings
- T2WI demonstrate edema
Imaging Recommendations
- Any lateral spread of C1 pillars on open mouth x-ray view requires CT
- CT details sites of fracture
- Thin section (1mm) cuts mandatory, reformations very helpful

Hangman's Fracture

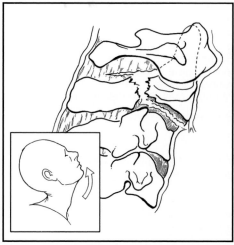

Hyperextension/distraction mechanism of Hangman's fracture is shown.

- Evaluate entire cervical spine (and even upper thoracic) as associated fractures occur in 33% of cases

Differential Diagnosis

<u>Pseudosubluxation</u>
- Seen in young children
- Affects multiple upper cervical levels
- Occurs on lateral x-ray view when mild flexion present
- No associated soft tissue swelling

Pathology

<u>General</u>
- General Path Comments
  - Classical hanging with knot in submental position produces complete disruption of disc and ligaments between C2 and C3
  - Sudden tearing of upper cord and brainstem by hyperextension and distraction
  - Traumatic TSA has different mechanism, similar results in bony spine
- Etiology-Pathogenesis
  - Traumatic TSA result from hyperextension with axial loading, or forced hyperflexion with compression in falls or MVAs
- Epidemiology
  - TSA represents 4-7% of all cervical fractures and/or dislocations
  - Isolated TSA represented 7% of all craniovertebal fractures in one series
  - Almost all modern cases represent sequelae of accidents rather than hanging

<u>Staging or Grading Criteria (If indicated)</u>
- Type I: Non-displaced, no angulation
- Type II: Significant angulation and translation
- Type III: Type II plus unilateral or bilateral facet dislocations

Hangman's Fracture

Clinical Issues

Presentation
- Pain upper neck after trauma
- Neurological sequelae uncommon in traumatic cases, as canal wide here and further decompressed by fracture
- Nevertheless, neurological sequelae occur in 25%
- Associated fractures elsewhere common, especially C1
- Vertebral artery injury may cause delayed neurological signs

Treatment
- Immobilization
- Fusion

Prognosis
- Depends on presence of neurological damage
- Accelerated degenerative changes

Selected References
1. Nunez DB et al: Cervical spine trauma: How much more do we learn by routinely using helical CT? Radiographics 16: 1307-18, 1996
2. Mivris SE et al: Hangman's fracture: radiologic assessment in 27 cases. Radiology 163: 713-7, 1987
3. Lee C et al: Fractures of the Craniovertebral junction associated with other fractures of the spine. AJNR 5: 775-81, 1984

Dens Fracture

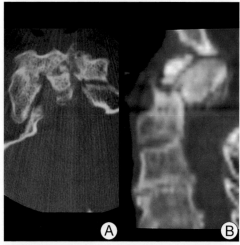

Axial CT image (A) shows bone disruption at the C2 level, but the plane of section is not parallel to the angulated fracture line, thus the sagittal reformation (B) best depicts the fracture at the base of the dens. Note bone sclerosis suggesting old fracture, and the calcification of the capsule posterior to the dens.

Key Facts
- Synonym: Odontoid fracture
- Definition: Traumatic bony disruption of the odontoid process
- Classic imaging appearance: Lucent linear defect through base of dens, with posterior displacement of it and arch of C1 relative to C2 body and arch
- Other key facts: Three patterns (Types I, II, III) are described
  - Type I: Avulsion of tip
  - Type II: Fracture at base of dens
  - Type III: Fracture extending into body of C2 (see drawing below)
- Fracture pattern dictates management
  - Type I fracture is an avulsion of the dens tip and considered stable, treated with simple immobilization
  - Type II is the most common, and most likely to go on to non-union; primary fusion may be indicated to prevent myelopathy
  - Type III involves the C2 body, nonunion is uncommon after treatment with traction followed by bracing

Imaging Findings
General Features
- Best imaging clue: Lateral and open mouth x-ray views depicting fracture line; posterior displacement and swelling of prevertebral soft tissue are strong supportive clues even when plain films are equivocal
CT Findings
- Comminuted bone at level of dens on axial views, fracture line on reformations, displacement at base of dens or tip of odontoid
MR Findings
- T1WI sagittal and coronal images best depict the disruption of bone contiguity, and degree of displacement. Marrow shows signal loss from edema in acute cases, normal signal indicates chronic non-union

Dens Fracture

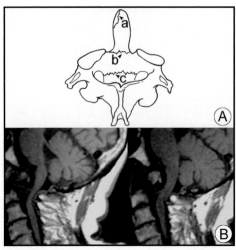

Drawing (A) depicts the three types of odontoid fracture. T1WI sagittal images (B) demonstrate Type II fracture. It is old and ununited (note lack of soft tissue swelling and marrow edema, the sclerotic fracture line showing low signal).

- T2WI serve to verify edematous marrow, and better depict associated soft tissue edema in prevertebral space (missing in chronic non-union)

Imaging Recommendations
- Plain x-rays (especially lateral and open-mouth views) initially suggest need for CT if any of the above mentioned clues are present
- Thin section (1mm) axial slices with bone reconstruction algorithm with fastest possible scan times for optimal reformation into sagittal and coronal planes
- MRI with T1WI in sagittal and coronal planes (3mm slices), T2WI in sagittal plane to evaluate canal size, cord injury. GRE imaging to detect blood in cord if myelopathy is present

Differential Diagnosis

Congenital Nonunion of Odontoid Tip (Os Odontoideum)
- Well-corticated ossification center above rudimentary dens
- No soft tissue swelling
- No history of trauma, or pain

Rheumatoid Arthritis-C1/C2 Subluxation
- Synovial proliferation erodes dens, leads to laxity and subluxation

Pathology

General
- Embryology-Anatomy
  - Three ossification centers form C2
  - Os odontoideum represents unfused ossification center atop dens C2
  - Type III fracture follows embryologic line of union between dens and body of C2
- Etiology-Pathogenesis
  - Caused by sudden forward or backward movement of the head, with the neck rigidly erect and articulations locked

o Osteoporosis in the elderly predisposes to Type II fracture and non-union

<u>Staging or Grading Criteria</u>
- The three patterns described are used for staging

Clinical Issues
<u>Presentation</u>
- Acute neck pain and possibly neurologic long tract signs
- Fluctuating long tract signs, spasticity may be the only presentation in older patients whose initial trauma was minor and not well diagnosed

<u>Natural History</u>
- Nonunion common in elderly without primary fusion. May stabilize by fibrous union with prolonged immobilization

<u>Treatment</u>
- Type I: Immobilization
- Type II: Primary fusion may be indicated
- Type III: Traction/bracing

<u>Prognosis</u>
- Chronic nonunion or fibrous union in elderly
- Fusion produces stability

Selected References
1. Brant-Zawadzki M et al:CT in the evaluation of spine trauma. AJR. 136: 369, 1981
2. Charlton OP et al: Roentgenographic evaluation of cervical spine trauma. JAMA. 242:1073-5, 1979
3. Anderson et al: Fractures of the odontoid process of the axis. J Bone and Joint Surg 56A: 1663-74, 1974

Rotatory Trauma with Facet Lock

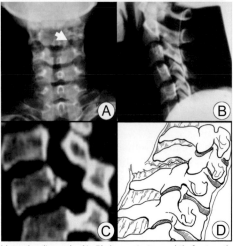

Frontral and lateral radiographs (A, B) demonstrate a subtle fracture (arrow) of left articular pillar of C4 and focal acute angulation at C4-5. Oblique CT reformation (C) demonstrates anterior facet subluxation of left C3 facet in respect to C4. (D) Mechanism of rotary trauma, resulting ligament tears and "jumped" facet.

Key Facts
- Synonym: Jumped facet(s)
- Definition: Traumatic disruption of cervical spinal structure (ligaments alone, or together with bony elements) leading to severe facet subluxation
- Classic imaging appearance: Malalignment of lateral masses (facets) on lateral x-ray with focal reversal of cervical spine contour (lordosis)
- Caused by rotatory forces during trauma
- Rotatory shear forces disrupt capsular, annular, longitudinal ligaments thus allowing even intact bony elements to easily sublux, damage neural tissue
  - Once facets "jump" each other and lock, the fracture is stable
  - Considerable traction is necessary to restore normal relationships
    - Neurological injury is common
    - Facet fracture fragments are often seen

Imaging Findings
General Features
- Best imaging clue: Focal malalignment of facet joints on lateral x-ray, accompanied by focal vertebral body (vb) angulation, rotation of spinous process off midline on AP view
CT Findings
- Axial views show reversal of normal relationship between facet of the lower vb with its upper neighbor
- Normally, the lower vb facet (superior facet) is **anteriorly** oriented in respect to its upper neighbor's inferior facet
MR Findings
- Demonstrates cord compromise, contusion when present
Imaging Recommendations
- 5 view cervical spine series starts the work-up

Rotatory Trauma with Facet Lock

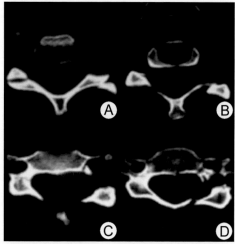

Consecutive axial CT (A-D) slices at C3-4 showing superior facet of C4 behind inferior facet of C3 with pedicle and laminar fracture. The free fragment floats behind C3 joint, explaining lack of significant vertebral body rotation (C, D).

- CT with thin axial sections and reformations recommended whenever a question is raised on x-rays, or if patient is severely injured or cannot cooperate
- Always evaluate the following relationships when examining C-spine trauma X-rays
    - Anterior vb alignment-should show gentle lordosis
    - Posterior edges of vb should parallel the anterior curve
    - Facets should align on lateral and oblique views
    - Posterior laminal line (point of junction of the laminae) should show the same gentle lordotic curve as that formed by the anterior and posterior vb edges on the lateral view
    - Prevertebral sof tissue should show ½ the thickness of AP vb diameter or less
    - AP x-ray should show regular spacing between spinous processes, all in midline
    - Disc space height loss can be a clue (in absence of degenerative changes)

Differential Diagnosis
- None

Pathology
General
- General Path Comments
    - Capsular ligaments provide considerable support to the relatively small facets of the cervical vbs
    - The almost horizontal articulation of these facets predisposes to easy subluxation once ligaments are torn

Rotatory Trauma with Facet Lock

Staging or Grading Criteria
- Facet subluxation may vary from mild (perched facets) with threat of further damage, to severe (locking) a fixed injury
- Fracture-subluxation combine to produce considerable instability

Clinical Issues
Presentation
- Severe neck pain, often associated with neurological compromise
Natural History
- Dictated by type and degree of neurological deficit
Treatment
- Traction
- Decompression and stabilization as necessary
- Fusion
Prognosis
- Mild cord contusion can regress
- Cord hematoma heralds grave prognosis

Selected References
1.   An HS et al: Cervical Spine Trauma. Spine. Vol 23:2713-29, 1998
2.   Brant-Zawadzki M et al: Trauma, Computed Tomography of the Spine and Spinal Cord. Newton TH, Potts DG, Clavadal Press, 149-86, 1983
3.   Holdsworth FW et al: Fractures, Dislocations and Fracture-Dislocations of the Spine. Journal of Bone and Joint Surgury. 45B: 6-20, 1963

Flexion/Extension Cervical Fx

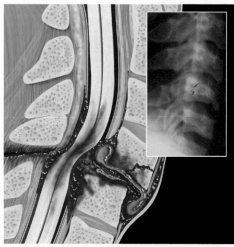

Sagittal graphic illustrates cervical fracture/subluxation with traumatic disc herniation, hemorrhage, and cord contusion. Lateral x-ray (inset) demonstrates wedge-compression fracture of C5, and pre-vertebral soft-tissue thickening; lucent line through arch is vaguely shown.

Key Facts
- Synonym: Whiplash fracture
- Definition: Vertebral body (vb) compression fracture and laminar fracture
- Classic imaging appearance: Compressed vb on x-ray with at least slight malalignment of C spine curvature, and associated pre-vertebral swelling
  - Can see abnormally asymmetric vertical separation of spinous processes on AP view, slight rotation of facets from true lateral on lateral view
    - CT defines components of fracture to best advantage

Imaging Findings
General Features
- Best imaging clue: Fragmented, wedged vb on lateral view with focal kyphosis

CT Findings
- Comminuted vb on axial view, with fractured arch (typically bilateral)
- Sagittal reformation shows vb compression, slight listhesis, pre-vertebral swelling

MR Findings
- T2WI demonstrate cord edema or hemorrhage, anterior longitudinal ligament disruption, and may show nuchal ligament injury
- GRE sequences most sensitive to blood in cord which heralds irreversible damage

Imaging Recommendations
- Must obtain CT once plain film findings suggest fracture
- CT often shows more fractures
- Thin section (1-3mm) cuts mandatory, reformations very helpful
- MR vital if neurologic signs present to evaluate cord injury, compression

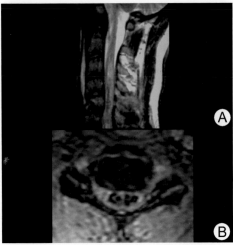

Sagittal T2WI (A) demonstrates hemorrhagic contusion of cord and vb compression. Axial GRE image (B) amplifies the low signal intensity of blood in the cord.

Differential Diagnosis
- None

Pathology
General
- General Path Comments
  - Disruption of anterior, middle and posterior columns of the spine causes mechanical instability
  - Neurological compromise subsequent to the injury may occur if unstable nature of fracture not recognized
  - Disc or bone fragment displacement can contribute to cord compression
- Etiology-Pathogenesis
  - Relatively small, flat, articular processes of C-spine exhibit almost horizontal articulation, with little overlap of articular surfaces
  - Ligaments (anterior, posterior longitudinal and capsular as well as ligamentum flavum and nuchae) provide considerable stability
  - Anatomy of C-spine predisposes to instability once ligaments are disrupted
  - Flexion, extension, rotation, and axial compression are the forces producing spine disruption
  - Flexion, compression and extension are often combined
  - Multiple, non-contiguous fractures may be seen in up to 25% of cases
  - Rotatory force can tear ligaments and produce instability, neurologic damage even without fracture, lead to facet subluxation, locking

Clinical Issues
Presentation
- Severe neck pain, with or without neurologic signs

Flexion/Extension Cervical Fx

- History of trauma with flexion/extension components and/or axial loading (e.g. diving)

Natural History
- Depends on presence and degree of neurologic compromise

Treatment
- If no neurological injury, treatment is aimed at immobilization (halo) and correction of any deformity
- If neurologic signs present, and compression found, acute decompression
- If cord is edematous, high dose steroids (first 24 hours)
- If cord demonstrates hemorrhage or transsection, immobilization to prevent further deformity

Prognosis
- Good if no neurologic damage, and stabilization achieved
- Accelerated degenerative disease may be seen
- Neurologic recovery can occur if only mild edema is seen in cord acutely
- Fixed neurologic deficit if cord shows hemorrhagic contusion
- Progression of fixed deficit superiorly if posttraumatic syrinx appears late

Selected References
1. Coin CG et al: Diving type injury of the cervical spine: Contribution of CT to management. J Comput Assist Tomogr. 3: 362-5, 1979
2. Penning L: Functional pathology of the cervical spine. Baltimore, Williams and Wilkins, 1968

Low Thoracic Distraction Fx

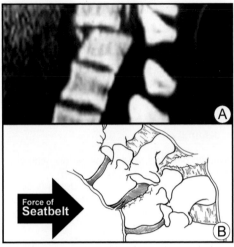

Sagittal CT (A) reformation with intrathecal dye (patient had paraplegia, MRI unavailable) shows canal malalignment and complete block indicating cord compression. Drawing (B) demonstrates the nature of the "seatbelt fracture".

Key Facts
- Synonym: Seatbelt fracture dislocation
- Definition: Vertebral body (vb) wedge compression and anterior displacement of spine above the fracture with facet subluxation
- Classic imaging appearance: Compressed anterior endplate or wedging of vb on x-ray with at least slight anterior subluxation
  - Lap belt restraint of torso during violent anterior displacement of upper body in car accident is a classic scenario
  - The orientation of thoracic curvature, the structure of rib cage translates most thoracic traumatic forces in to flexion component
  - Thoracic-lumbar junctional region is the second most common location (after cervical) where neurological injury accompanies fracture (30%)
    - CT defines components of fracture to best advantage
    - MRI best for evaluating associated neurologic injury, intrathecal dye necessary with CT if MRI unavailable

Imaging Findings
General Features
- Best imaging clue: Wedged vb on lateral view with focal kyphosis, some degree of anterior displacement of upper vb, separation of spinous processes
CT Findings
- Fragmented anterior endplate of vb on axial view, with diminished or absent facet overlap (typically bilateral)
- Sagittal reformations show vb compression, anterior slippage of vb above, and perched or jumped facets
MR Findings
- T2WI demonstrate cord compression if any, edema or hemorrhage, ligament disruption, and microtrabecular disruption of vb

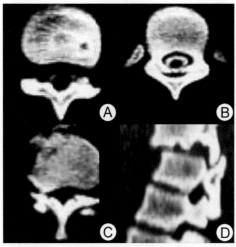

Consecutive axial CT (A-C) slices show the "naked" inferior facets of T11, upwardly and anteriorly displaced from the superior facets of T12. Note the interruption of the thecal dye collar at the level of fracture. Sagittal reformation (D) in the plane of the facet joint shows the jumped facets.

- GRE sequences most sensitive to blood in cord which heralds irreversible damage

<u>Imaging Recommendations</u>
- Must obtain CT once plain film findings suggest fracture
- Thin section (1-3mm) cuts mandatory, reformations very helpful, particularly in sagittal midline, and along vertical axis of facets
- MR vital if neurologic signs present to evaluate cord injury, compression

Differential Diagnosis
- None

Pathology
<u>General</u>
- General Path Comments
  - Disruption of anterior, middle and posterior columns of the spine causes mechanical instability
  - Neurological compromise subsequent to the injury is caused by the canal compromise at time of subluxation
  - Disc or bone fragment displacement can contribute to cord compression
- Etiology-Pathogenesis
  - Considerable force needed to displace the broad, coronally overlapped thoracic facets
  - Ligaments (anterior, posterior longitudinal and capsular as well as ligamenta flavum) provide considerable stability, are torn with this mechanism
  - Neurological compromise common in this injury

Low Thoracic Distraction Fx

Clinical Issues

Presentation
- Severe pain, often with paraplegia, bowel and bladder signs
- History of deceleration trauma with flexion
- Natural History: Depends on presence and degree of neurologic compromise

Treatment
- If no neurological injury, treatment is aimed at correction of deformity with traction and stabilization with Harrington rod fusion
- If neurologic signs present, and compression found, acute decompression
- If cord is edematous, high-dose steroids (first 24 hours) may be used

Prognosis
- Good if no neurologic damage, and stabilization achieved
- Accelerated degenerative disease may be seen
- Neurologic recovery can occur if only mild edema is seen in cord acutely
- Fixed neurologic deficit if cord shows hemorrhagic contusion

Selected References
1. Brant-Zawadzki M et al: High-resolution CT of thoracolumbar fractures. AJNR 3:69-72, 1982
   Contribution of CT to management. J Comput Assist Tomogr. 3: 362-65, 1979
2. Burke DC et al: The management of thoracic and thoracolumbar injuries of the spine with neurologic involvement. J Bone and Joint Surg 58B:72-5, 1976
3. Rogers LF: The Roentgenographic appearance of transverse fractures of the spine: the seatbelt fracture. AJR 111: 844-6, 1971

Burst Fracture

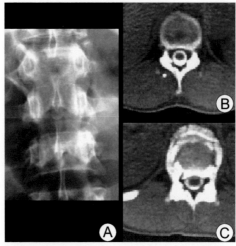

AP plain flim (A) shows widened pedicles. Axial CT slice (B,C) following intrathecal contrast shows multiple vertebral body fracture planes and fragment retropulsion into spinal canal, but does not suggest cord impingement

Key Facts
- Synonym: Unstable compression fracture
- Definition: Comminuted fracture of vertebral body (vb) extending through both superior and inferior endplates
- Classic imaging appearance: Compressed vb, widened pedicles on AP view, stellate pattern of fracture lines on axial CT
- Unstable fracture despite intact posterior elements
  - Middle column disruption produces instability
    - Retropulsed bone may compromise conus, cauda equina

Imaging Findings
General Features
- Best imaging clue: Compressed lower thoracic or upper lumbar vb with fractured endplates and widened pedicles on trauma x-rays
CT Findings
- Comminution of vb, retropulsed posterior fragments
MR Findings
- Vb height and signal loss on T1WI, hyperintense vb on T2WI
- May see prevertebral hematoma, blood or disc in canal
- May see cord contusion at L1 or above
Imaging Recommendations
- Always obtain CT if pedicular widening accompanies VB compression
- Thin section axial slices with sagittal reformations, bone and soft tissue windows
- MR vital if neurologic symptoms/signs present

Differential Diagnosis
Benign Compression Fracture
- Typically anterior wedge compression
- No endplate-to-endplate comminution

Burst Fracture

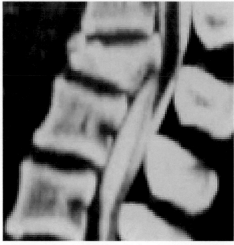

Sagittal reconstruction of post myelogram CT demonstrates compromise of canal is greater than suggested by the axial slice, the original plane of the axial sections was not parallel to the plane compromising canal.

- No retropulsion of fragments or pedicular widening

Pathologic Compression Fracture
- Soft tissue mass replacing major portion of vb on MR
- No branching fracture lines on CT

Pathology
General
- General Path Comments
  - Typically due to vertical force trauma (jumping, landing on buttock)

Clinical Issues
Presentation
- Focal back pain after trauma with vertical force component
- Radiculopathy or myelopathy (depending on level) may be present

Natural History
- Self-limited unless neurologic injury becomes permanent

Treatment
- Surgical stabilization and (if needed) canal decompression
  - Bed rest may be sufficient with immobilization if comminution is minimal

Prognosis
- Good, unless permanent cord or nerve root injury
  - May have column deformity (kyphosis) in severe cases

Selected References
1. Ballock RT et al: Can burst fractures be predicted from plain radiographs? J Bone Joint Surg Br. 74: 147 1992
2. McAffee PC et al: The unstable burst fracture. Spine 7: 365-73, 1982
3. Holdsworth FW: Fractures, dislocations, and fracture-dislocations of the spine. J Bone and Joint Surg Br. 45: 6-20, 1963

Sacral Insufficiency Fracture

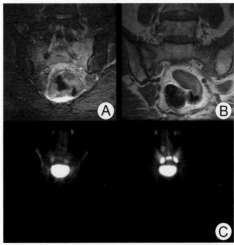

Oblique coronal fat suppressed T2WI (A) demonstrates bilateral sacral marrow hyperintensities. Corresponding hypointensity is seen in the left sacral ala on coronal T1WI (B), which also reveals a right sacral alar fracture. The "H" shaped pattern of uptake on bone scintigraphy is present in another patient (C).

Key Facts
- Definition: Sacral fracture resulting from normal physiological stress on demineralized bone with decreased elastic resistance
- Classic imaging appearance
  - "H" shaped pattern of increased radiotracer uptake in the sacrum on bone scintigraphy
  - Patchy and/or curvilinear signal alteration on MRI, hypointense on T1WI, hyperintense on T2WI, through sacral alae
  - Bilateral sacral alar patchy sclerosis parallel to the sacroiliac joints on plain film and CT
- Other key facts
  - High clinical suspicion required to make the diagnosis
  - Signs and symptoms mimic
    - Degenerative disc disease
    - Spinal stenosis
    - Vertebral compression fracture
    - Hip arthritis
  - Approximately half of the plain films will be normal at the time of presentation
  - MRI highly sensitive for marrow edema
  - May be unilateral
  - Concomitant vertebral and pubic insufficiency fractures

Imaging Findings
General Features
- Best imaging clue: Bilateral or unilateral sacral edema parallel to the sacroiliac joint(s) on MRI
CT Findings
- Bony sclerosis

Sacral Insufficiency Fracture

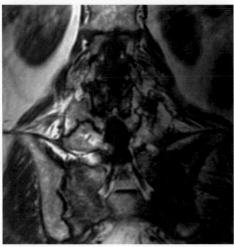

Sacral insufficiency fracture. Oblique coronal T1WI in another patient demonstrates bilateral sacral marrow hypointensities (L > R) parallel to the sacroiliac joints.

- Fracture lines may or may not extend to anterior sacral cortex

MR Findings
- Patchy bilateral or unilateral sacral edema
  o Hypointense on T1WI
  o Hyperintense on T2WI
- Parallel to sacroiliac joint(s)
- Presence of fracture line(s)
- Lack of bony expansion or soft tissue mass

Plain Film Findings
- Approximately half will be normal at the time of presentation
- Osteopenia
- Vertical band(s) of sclerosis parallel to the sacroiliac joint(s)
- Lucent fracture line(s)

Bone Scintigraphy Findings
- Bilateral or unilateral sacral radiotracer uptake with or without a horizontal component
- Characteristic "H" shaped pattern of radiotracer uptake only present in 19% of the cases

Imaging Recommendations
- Gadolinium-enhanced axial T1WI or fat suppressed sequences may better delineate the fracture line
- Imaging in the oblique coronal plane also helps to visualize the fracture line

Differential Diagnosis
Sacral Metastases
- More discrete in morphology
- Random distribution
- Invasion of adjacent soft tissue, neural foramina
- Other sites involved

Sacral Insufficiency Fracture

Primary Sacral Neoplasm
- Large and solitary
- Bony expansion and cortical breakthrough
- Soft-tissue component

Pathology
General
- General Path Comments
  o Underlying abnormal bony mineralization
- Etiology-Pathogenesis
  o Predisposing factors
    ▪ Osteoporosis
    ▪ Rheumatoid arthritis
    ▪ Renal osteodystrophy
    ▪ Endogenous or exogenous corticosteroid excess
    ▪ Radiation therapy
    ▪ Other causes of osteopenia
    ▪ Paget's disease
  o Minor trauma
    ▪ Often elicited after the diagnosis
  o No precipitating event in many instances
- Epidemiology
  o Incidence from 0.14% to 1.8%
  o Seventh and eighth decades of life
  o More common in women
Microscopic Features
- Bony necrosis
- Bone marrow fibrosis

Clinical Issues
Presentation
- Acute or subacute pain
  o Low back
  o Buttock
  o Exacerbated by activity
  o Relieved by rest
- Radicular symptoms
Treatment
- Bed rest
- Analgesics
- Physical therapy
Prognosis
- Favorable outcome
- Asymptomatic in 2 weeks to 24 months
- May be limited by co-morbidities

Selected References
1. Grangier C et al: Role of MRI in the diagnosis of insufficiency fractures of the sacrum and acetabular roof. Skeletal Radio 26:517-24, 1997
2. Peh WC et al: Imaging of pelvic insufficiency fractures. Radiographics 16:335-48, 1996
3. Grasland A et al: Sacral insufficiency fractures: an easily overlooked cause of back pain in elderly women. Arch Intern Med 156:668-74, 1996

Jefferson Fracture

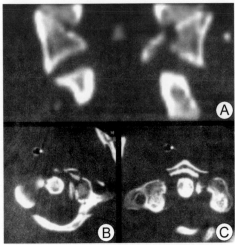

Axial CT (B,C) shows multiple defects of C1 arch. Coronal reformation (A) depicts C1 pillars laterally displaced from those of C2. Avulsed fragment off the inner left C1 pillar-the attachment for the transverse ligament-suggestsC1-C2 instability at C1-C2.

Key Facts
- Synonym: Atlas burst fracture
- Definition: Compression fracture of the C1 arch
- Classic imaging appearance: Bony defects of C1 arch on lateral x-ray, displacement of **both** lateral masses of C1 laterally from those of C2 on open mouth view
  - Can see separation between dens and anterior arch of C1
  - Soft tissue swelling anterior to C1 common
- CT defines components of fracture to best advantage
- May see various patterns of arch disruption

Imaging Findings
General Features
- Best imaging clue: Lateral displacement of articular masses of C1 from those of C2 on open-mouth view
CT Findings
- Multiple fractures of C1 arch typical
- Both anterior and posterior arch fractures are seen only in minority
- Posterior arch fractured more often than anterior
- Lateral masses alone may be fractured
- A single site of arch fracture may occur
- Look for avulsion of inner pillar at insertion of transverse ligament
MR Findings
- T2WI demonstrate edema
Imaging Recommendations
- Any lateral spread of C1 pillars on open-mouth x-ray view requires CT
- CT details sites of fracture
- Thin section (1mm) cuts mandatory, reformations very helpful
- Evaluate entire cervical spine (and even upper thoracic) as associated fractures occur in 24% of cases

Jefferson Fracture

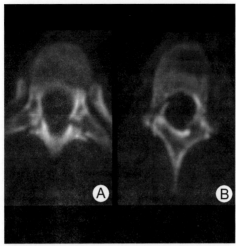

Axial CT (A,B) demonstrates associated posterior element fractures at T3, due to the axial compression which caused the Jefferson fracture.

Differential Diagnosis

Pseudospread of the Atlas in Children
- Common finding in many children 3 months to four years of age evaluated for minor trauma
- Seen in 90% or more of two year olds
- Caused by disparity in growth rates of the atlas and axis
- Jefferson fracture rare in young children – greater plasticity, synchondroses of C1 arch serve as "buffer"

Congenital Clefts, Malformations of Atlas
- May show 1-2 mm offset of C1 pillars from those of C2
- Clefts found in 4% of posterior arches, 0.1% of anterior arches
- 97% of posterior clefts are midline, 3% through sulcus of vertebral artery
- Various deficiencies of arch development can be seen
- Most are partial hemiaplasias of posterior arch
- Clefts and congenital defects show smooth or well-corticated edges

Rotational Malalignment of Atlas, Axis Pillars
- Generally seen unilaterally, with rotation and abduction of head

Pathology

General
- General Path Comments
    - Rough-edge fragmentation of C1 arch at one or more sites
    - Typically a stable fracture, unless transverse ligament avulsed, more than 7 mm offset a clue to such avulsion and instability
    - Combined fractures occur, especially with C2
- Etiology-Pathogenesis
    - Axial compressive force applied to skull's vertex
    - Force transmitted down through occipital condyles onto C1 pillars with head and neck rigidly erect
- Epidemiology
    - C1 fractures represent 6% of all vertebral injuries

Jefferson Fracture

- o One-third of C1 fractures are the classic burst Jefferson fracture
- o Rare in infants and young children

Clinical Issues

Presentation
- Upper neck pain
- Often missed on plain films

Natural History
- Stable fracture with healing in majority of isolated cases

Treatment
- Immobilization, fusion if gross instability

Selected References
1. Harris JH: The cervicocranium: its radiographic assessment. Radiology 218:337-51, 2001
2. Gehwiler JA et al: Malformations of the atlas simulating the Jefferson fracture. AJNR 4:187-90, 1983
3. Jefferson G: Fracture of the atlas vertebra. Report of four cases and a review of those previously recorded. Br J Surg 7:407-11, 1920

Central Cord Syndrome

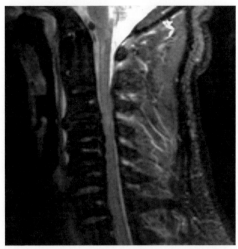

Sagittal T2WI with fat saturation of the cervical spine demonstrates central stenosis from C3 to C6. Subtle T2 hyperintensity is present in the cord from C3 to C4. Prevertebral soft tissue T2 hyperintensity is reflective of hyperextension injury.

Key Facts
- Synonym(s): Spinal cord concussion, transient traumatic cord apraxia
- Definition: Immediate complete posttraumatic paralysis with variable sensory loss, largely preserved proprioception and sense of vibration
- Classic imaging appearance: Congenital and/or acquired canal stenosis, normal or slightly edematous cord on MRI, effaced CSF sac
- Encompasses a spectrum of clinical posttraumatic cord syndromes which resolve to considerable degree within hours to days
  - Spinal cord concussion
    - Completely reversible
    - Seen most often in athletes
    - Functional rather than mechanical interruption of neuronal activity
  - Anterior cervical cord syndrome
    - Immediate complete paralysis, altered sensation
    - Preserved vibratory/positional sense
    - Almost complete recovery
    - Slight residual spasticity
  - Posterior cervical cord syndrome
    - Pain and paresthesias in neck, upper arms and trunk
    - Symmetric and burning sensation
    - May have mild paresis of arms

Imaging Findings
General Features
- Best imaging clue: Spinal stenosis, congenital and/or acquired
CT Findings
- May be normal or show only stenotic canal
- Can see fracture or subluxation
- Can see disc bulging or protrusion/extrusion

Central Cord Syndrome

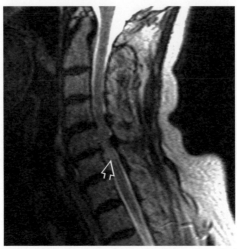

Sagittal T2WI (fat sat) demonstrates central stenosis from C3 to C6. Note effaced CSF, subtle T2 cord hyperintensity (arrow).

<u>MR Findings</u>
- Normal or slightly tumescent cord
- Without or with slight hyperintensity on T2WI
- Stenotic canal, or
- Disc bulging/protrusion/extrusion

Differential Diagnosis
<u>Cord Contusion</u>
- Generally much slower recovery
- Greater residual deficit
- Swollen edematous cord on MRI
<u>Cord Hematoma</u>
- No or little recovery long term
- Low signal from blood on T2WI and GRE

Pathology
<u>General</u>
- General Path Comments
  - o Spectrum of changes seen in experimental models
  - o Cord may be normal - kinetic energy reversibly blocks impulse transmission
  - o May see slight edema
  - o Axonal stretching analogous to "shear injury" in brain?
- Etiology-Pathogenesis
  - o True cord concussion is fully reversible in < 72 hours
  - o Most often seen in young athletes
  - o May have normal canal
  - o Can affect thoracolumbar junction (conus)
  - o Central cord syndrome associated with spinal stenosis

- Abnormal Torg's ratio (AP dimension of spinal canal to vertebral body less than 0.8)
  - o Generally seen in hyperextension injury
  - o Spur, disc or ligamentous ossification predispose to it
- Epidemiology
  - o One study estimated that 1.3 of every 10,000 US football players sustained it
  - o Up to 25% of traumatic paralysis associated with restricted canal

Clinical Issues

Presentation
- Immediate paralysis/paresis with varying sensory loss after trauma

Natural History
- Complete resolution to slight residual weakness and spasticity

Treatment
- Initial stabilization if spinal instability suspected
- Decompression if focal stenosis
- Steroid therapy in first 24 hours may have a role

Prognosis
- Generally complete or near complete reversal of the acute paralysis

Selected References
1.   An HS: Cervical Spine trauma. Spine 23:2713-29, 1998
2.   Zwimpfer TJ et al: Spinal cord concussion. J Neurosurg 72:894-900, 1990
3.   Torg JS et al: Neurapraxia of the cervical spinal cord with transient quadriplegia. J Bone Joint Surg (Am)68:1354-70, 1986

Syrinx

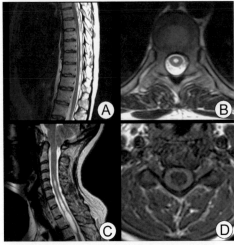

Idiopathic syrinx: Sagittal and axial T2WI (A, B) show characteristic central fusiform dilatation of central cord. Chiari I: Sagittal T2WI and axial T1WI (C, D) show tonsillar ectopia with associated cervical syrinx.

Key Facts
- Synonym(s): Syringomyelia, Syringohydromyelia
- Definition: Cystic spinal cord cavity that may (hydromyelia) or may not (syringomyelia) communicate with the central spinal cord canal
  - Artificial distinction – many use term syringohydromyelia
- Classic imaging appearance: Cystic, expansile lesion of central spinal cord
- Syrinx may be primary or secondary
- Main imaging goal is to exclude associated or causative lesions

Imaging Findings
General Features
- Longitudinal spinal cord cleft with CSF imaging characteristics
- Best imaging clue: Expansile cord with dilated central cystic cavity
CT Findings
- Cord expansion with central CSF density spinal cord cavitation
  - May be difficult to appreciate central cavity on unenhanced imaging
  - Delayed CT myelography imaging best demonstrates central canal
- May see posterior vertebral body scalloping in longstanding lesions
MR Findings
- Sagittal images best demonstrate lesion extent
  - Syrinx frequently has a fusiform "beaded" appearance
- Axial images confirm lesion location and clarify relationship to adjacent anatomical structures
- Contrast is essential to exclude neoplastic syrinx
  - No syrinx enhancement seen in idiopathic non-neoplastic cases
Other Modality Findings
- Sagittal 2D cine phase contrast (PC) CSF flow studies may show abnormal CSF dynamics across tonsils (Chiari I) or other putative causative lesions
- Plain film – central canal widening, shoulder atrophic neuroarthropathy

Syrinx

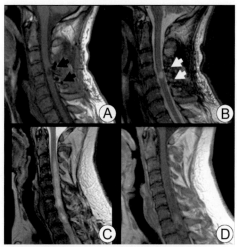

Posttraumatic syrinx: Sagittal T1WI and T2WI (A, B) reveal focal syrinx at level of repaired fracture-dislocation (arrows denotes posterior fixation hardware). Cord astrocytoma with syrinx: Sagittal T2WI, enhanced T1WI (C, D) demonstrate central cavitation and enhancing mass.

Imaging Recommendations
- MR imaging is modality of choice
  - Both T1WI and T2WI sequences should be acquired
- Syrinx best appreciated on axial images; sagittal sequence useful for approximating craniocaudal extent
- Contrast essential to exclude neoplasm
- Consider cine PC CSF flow study if suspect anatomical obstruction to CSF flow (e.g. tonsillar ectopia or arachnoid adhesions)

Differential Diagnosis
Ventriculus Terminalis
- Asymptomatic (normal) dilatation of central canal in terminal cord/conus
Myelomalacia
- Cord volume loss, gliosis
- Do not see CSF signal central cavitation on T1WI
Cystic Spinal Cord Tumor
- Astrocytoma, ependymoma, hemangioblastoma
- Cord expansion; nearly always have enhancing component

Pathology
General
- General Path Comments
  - Longitudinally oriented CSF-filled cavity with surrounding gliosis
    - Hydromyelia: Central canal dilatation
    - Syringomyelia: Cavity is lateral to or independent of central canal
    - Most cases show features of both on pathologic exam (e.g. syringohydromyelia)
  - Medullary extension is termed syringobulbia
  - Central canal patency may determine syrinx extent

- o CSF diastolic flow characteristics may determine cyst size and its biological behavior
- Etiology-Pathogenesis
  - o Primary: Idiopathic or in conjunction with Chiari I or II malformation, spinal dysraphism, diastematomyelia
  - o Secondary:Tumor, inflammatory (arachnoiditis, SAH), or trauma
- Etiology is actively debated; two currently most popular theories are not mutually exclusive
  - o Subarachnoid space abnormality drives CSF into vulnerable cord through perivascular spaces
  - o Cord destruction is related to primary cord disease process
- Epidemiology
  - o Primary syrinx usually occurs in younger patients
  - o Secondary syrinx may occur at any age; timing of appearance may be determined by behavior of primary inciting disease

Microscopic Features
- Tubular spinal cord cavitation surrounded by dense glial fibril wall
- Initially central; frequently eccentric
  - o Larger lesions may extend into the anterior commissure, posterior horn

Clinical Issues

Presentation
- Usual presentation in adults
- Uncommon in childhood
  - o Most childhood cases are either simple hydromyelia or associated with Chiari malformation
  - o More likely than adults to present with scoliosis
- "Cloak–like" pain and temperature sensory loss with preservation of position sense, proprioception, and light touch
- Subsequently develop distal upper extremity weakness (especially hand) followed by gait instability
- Cranial neuropathies implicate syringobulbia

Treatment
- Address underlying causative etiology when possible
- Drain syrinx with indwelling catheter when it is not possible to restore normal cord CSF dynamics by addressing cause

Prognosis
- Variable; dependant on underlying etiology

Selected References
1. Brugieres P et al: CSF flow measurement in syringomyelia. AJNR 21(10): 1785-92, 2000
2. Castillo M: Further explanations for the formation of syringomyelia: back to the drawing table. AJNR 21(10): 1778-9, 2000
3. Fischbein NJ et al: The "presyrinx" state: a reversible myelopathic condition that may precede syringomyelia. AJNR 20(1): 7-20, 1999

Vertebral Dissection

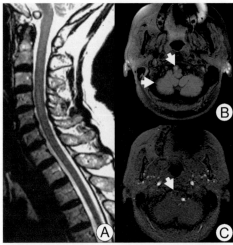

Sagittal T2 of the cervical spine (A) demonstrates subtle cord ischemia at C4 and C5. Axial T1WI with fat saturation (B) reveals a hyperintense hematoma filling the right distal intracranial vertebral artery (arrow). On 2D TOF MRA (C), there is corresponding loss of flow related signal (arrow).

Key Facts
- Definition: Hemorrhage into damaged vessel wall with subsequent stenosis or pseudoaneurysm
- Classic imaging appearance: Enlarged external diameter of the artery with intramural crescentic T1 hyperintensity
- Carotid and vertebral dissection responsible for 2% of all cerebrovascular accidents
  - Causes 10% to 25% of all infarcts in young and middle-aged patients
- Posttraumatic neurological symptoms may be delayed
  - More than one week after the initial injury
- 3D time-of-flight MR angiography
  - Less sensitive for vertebral artery dissection compared to conventional angiography
  - Equally sensitive for carotid artery dissection

Imaging Findings
General Features
- Best imaging clue: T1 hyperintensity surrounding a diminished flow void
MR Findings
- Intramural hematoma
  - Hyperintense on fat suppressed T1WI and T2WI
    - May be isointense initially
  - Crescentic, circumferential, or filling the entire lumen
  - May enhance after intravenous gadolinium
  - May spiral along the artery
- Normal or narrowed flow void
- Thin, curvilinear, hypointense intimal flap
- Subarachnoid hemorrhage may be present if intracranial extension (10%)
- MR angiography

Vertebral Dissection

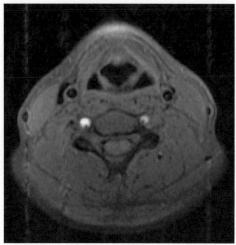

Axial T1WI with fat saturation in another patient shows bilateral vertebral crescentic intramural hematomas with narrowed flow void.

- o Intramural hematoma intermediate signal intensity between flow-related enhancement and surrounding soft tissue
    - ▪ May be isointense to soft tissue
- o Flow enhancement in pseudoaneurysm

<u>Conventional Angiography Findings</u>
- Most common at the C1-2 vertebral bodies
- Smoothly or slightly irregular tapered luminal narrowing
    - o Slight stenosis -> "string sign" -> total occlusion
- Pseudoaneurysm (25% to 35%)
- Intimal flap (10%) and double lumen
- Branch vessel occlusion from embolization

<u>Imaging Recommendations</u>
- Axial T1WI with fat saturation through the neck

Differential Diagnosis

<u>Atherosclerotic Disease</u>
- At the vertebral artery origin
- More focal
- No intramural hematoma

<u>Fibromuscular Disease</u>
- Can present with focal narrowing on conventional angiogram
- Vertebral artery involvement (7%) less common than carotid (85%)
- No intramural hematoma

Pathology

<u>General</u>
- Genetics
    - o Connective tissue disorder predisposing to spontaneous dissection
        - ▪ Present in up to 25% of patients with dissection
        - ▪ Ehlers-Danlos syndrome, Marfan's syndrome, autosomal dominant polycystic kidney disease

- o Other arteriopathies
    - ▪ Fibromuscular dysplasia (15%)
    - ▪ Cystic medial necrosis
- • Embryology-Anatomy
    - o Sites of greater mobility most susceptible to injury
        - ▪ Proximal: Between the origin in the subclavian artery to C6 transverse processes
        - ▪ Distal: Cranial to C2 transverse processes, before entering the dura
- • Etiology-Pathogenesis
    - o Spontaneous
    - o Hypertension: Primary or drug-induced, including over-the-counter, e.g. ephedrine
    - o Major penetrating or blunt trauma
    - o Trivial trauma (coughing, sneezing, roller-coaster ride, chiropractic)
        - ▪ Prolonged or sudden neck hyperextension or rotation may be a precipitating factor
    - o Intimal tear or ruptured vasa vasorum -> intramural hematoma -> stenosis or pseudoaneurysm -> thrombus formation -> emboli
    - o Underlying atherosclerosis uncommon
- • Epidemiology
    - o Estimate of 1 to 1.5 per 100,000
    - o Affecting all ages, peak in the fifth decade of life

Microscopic Features
- • Hematoma within the tunica media of the vessel wall
    - o Compressing the intima, distending the adventitia

Clinical Issues

Presentation
- • May affect multiple vessels
    - o Horner's syndrome if carotid artery involved
- • Unilateral or bilateral occipital headache and posterior neck pain
- • Unilateral arm pain or weakness
- • Brainstem infarct
    - o Lateral medullary syndrome of Wallenberg
- • Cerebellar or posterior cerebral artery territory ischemia

Natural History
- • Spontaneously healing or recanalization in most cases

Treatment
- • Anticoagulation, unless contraindications present
- • If persistent ischemia or recurrent embolic events
    - o Surgical ligation or endovascular occlusion
    - o Percutaneous angioplasty

Prognosis
- • Resolution or significant improvement of stenosis in 90% within the first 2 to 3 months
- • Recurrence rate of 8%, 50% within the first month

Selected References
1. Schievink WI: Spontaneous dissection of the carotid and vertebral arteries. N Engl J Med 344:898-906, 2001
2. Provenzale JM: Dissection of the internal carotid and vertebral arteries: Imaging features. AJR 165: 1099-104, 1995
3. Levy C et al: Carotid and vertebral artery dissection: Three-dimensional time-of-flight MR angiography and MR imaging versus conventional angiography. Radiology 190:97-103, 1994

Lumbar Fracture with Dural Tear

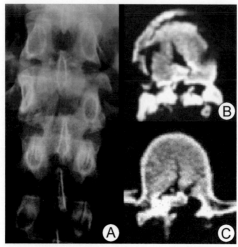

AP plain film (A) demonstrates widened pedicles, vertical arch defect and compression of L1. Axial CT slices (B, C) demonstrate subluxed T12/L1 facets due to "sprung" L1, fractured arch of L1 and parent vertebral body.

Key Facts
- Synonym: Compression Fracture
- Definition: Vertebral body (vb) compression fracture and laminar fracture with associated dural tear
- Classic imaging appearance: Compressed vb on x-ray with arch fracture, widened pedicles

Imaging Findings
General Features
- Best imaging clue: Wedged vb on lateral view with focal kyphosis, widened pedicles on AP view with vertical fracture through laminae

CT Findings
- Endplate fragmentation on axial view, with fractured arch (typically cleaved)
  - Sagittal reformation shows vb compression, slight listhesis
  - CT defines components of fracture to best advantage
    - Intrathecal dye needed to verify dural tear-shows leak
    - Cauda equina entrapment due to herniation of nerve roots (NR)

MR Findings
- T2WI demonstrate canal-conus relationship, may show CSF leak
- GRE sequences most sensitive to blood in conus

Imaging Recommendations
- Must obtain CT once plain film findings suggest fracture
  - Thin section (1-3mm) cuts mandatory, reformations very helpful
  - Intrathecal dye useful to demonstrate dural tear
  - Dural tear warns surgeon to look for NR if posterior fusion planned
- MR vital if myelopathy signs present to evaluate cord injury, compression

Differential Diagnosis
- None

Lumbar Fracture with Dural Tear

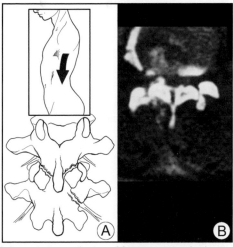

Drawing (A) demonstrates mechanism of fracture causing dural tear. Reformatted post myelogram CT (B) shows leaking dye verifying dural tear.

Pathology

General
- General Path Comments
  - Disruption of vb, arch
  - Dural tear, arch fracture allow NR to escape confines of canal
- Etiology-Pathogenesis
  - Severe compression force on lumbar region when it is rigid or extended
  - NRs may become entrapped within arch fragments, or extend into soft tissues beyond arch

Clinical Issues

Presentation
- Severe back pain, with or without radiculopathy
- History of trauma with vertical force applied during lumbar extension, i.e. axial loading

Natural History
- Depends on presence and degree of neurologic compromise

Treatment
- Treatment is aimed at immobilization, fixation (rods) and closing dura
  - If neurologic signs present, care taken not to transect NR on approach

Prognosis
- Good if no neurologic damage, and stabilization achieved
- Accelerated degenerative disease may be seen

Selected References
1. Morris RE et al: Traumatic dural tears: CT diagnosis using metrizamide. Radiology 152: 443-6, 1984
2. Brant-Zawadzki M et al: High-resolution CT of thoracolumbar fractures. AJNR 3: 69-72,1982
3. Miller CA et al: Impaction Fracture of the lumbar vertebrae with dural tear. J. Neurosurg 53:765-8, 1980

DEGENERATIVE

Schmorl's Node

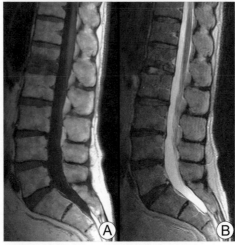

Sagittal T1WI (A) and T2WI (B) demonstrate disc material herniated through the inferior endplate of L1 into the vertebral body. Surrounding edema is better seen on T1WI (A) as marrow hypointensity.

Key Facts
- Synonym: Intravertebral disc herniation
- Definition: Cartilaginous nodes within vertebral body (VB) representing vertical disc extension through areas of weakness in the VB endplate
- Classic imaging appearance: Contour defect within endplate, extending from disc space into VB spongiosa with well-corticated margins on plain films
- Common incidental finding
- Rarely symptomatic

Imaging Findings
General Features
- Best imaging clue: Focal invagination of endplate by disc material surrounded by normal, corticated bone

CT Findings
- Axial CT shows well-circumscribed, scalloped, soft-tissue defect surrounded by VB cancellous bone with sclerotic margins; reformations demonstrate contiguity with parent disc space
- Schmorl's node may calcify

MR Findings
- T1WI show disc material contiguous with parent imploding into normal marrow; acute cases may show hypointense zone of edema in marrow
- T2 signal intensity of intravertebral disc matches parent interspace; zone of edema in acute cases may show considerable extent
- Peripheral contrast enhancement in subacute stage, diffuse marrow enhancement in acute stage

Other Modality Findings
- Nuclear imaging may show technetium uptake

Imaging Recommendations
- Analyze contiguity with parent disc on all sequences

Schmorl's Node

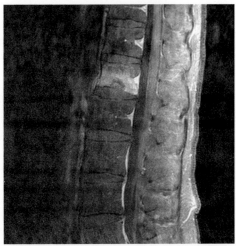

Sagittal post-gadolinium T1WI with fat saturation shows diffuse marrow enhancement surrounding the Schmorl's node.

Differential Diagnosis

Acute Compression Fracture
- Simulates diffuse edema of acute Schmorl's node, may in fact predispose to its ultimate formation; lacks imploded disc nodule within abnormal marrow

Focal Metastasis
- May be difficult to exclude from acute Schmorl's node if isolated
- Does not show contiguity with parent disc or its signal intensity

Pathology

General
- General Path Comments
  - Schmorl's node represents cartilaginous disc tissue with degenerative or inflammatory changes, and subsequent sclerotic response of trabecular condensation and thickening
    - The pathologic staging mirrors that of a focal endplate fracture
    - The typical Schmorl's node is a healed focal endplate fracture
- Embryology-Anatomy
  - Anulus actually biomechanically more resistant to mechanical failure than endplate in young individuals
  - Focal weakness of endplate predisposes to Schmorl's node formation
  - Associated with endplate weakening of Scheuermann's disease
- Etiology-Pathogenesis
  - Typically repetitive stress of gravity on weakened endplate
  - Acute axial traumatic load can lead to Schmorl's node formation with focal back pain
  - Osteoporosis, neoplasm, and infection can weaken endplate
- Epidemiology
  - Seen in up to 75% of all normal spines
  - Typically the inferior endplate is involved
  - Thoracolumbar spine most commonly affected

Schmorl's Node

Clinical Issues

Presentation
- Incidental finding
- Low back pain if traumatically induced

Natural History
- Self-limited

Treatment
- Observational, with pain management in symptomatic cases

Prognosis
- Good, unless systemic osteoporosis leads to recurrent compression fractures

Selected References
1. Wagner AL et al: Relationship of Schmorl's nodes to vertebral body endplate fractures and acute endplate disc extrusions. AJNR 21: 276-81, 2000
2. Stabler A et al: MR imaging of enhancing intraosseous disc herniation (Schmorl's nodes). AJR. 168: 933-8, 1997
3. Resnick D et al: Intravertebral disc herniations: Cartilaginous (Schmorl's) nodes. Radiology 126: 57-65, 1978

Disc Bulge

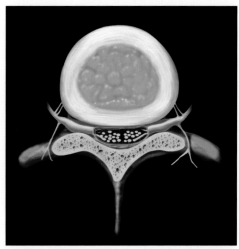

Axial illustration demonstrates a diffusely bulging anulus, flattening the thecal sac.

Key Facts
- Definition: Generalized extension of disc material beyond the edges of vertebral ring apophyses
- Classic imaging appearance: Circumferential disc "expansion" beyond the margin of vertebral endplate
- > 50% of the disc circumference
- Short radius of extension
  o Usually < 3 mm
- Often associated with degenerative disc disease
- Other causes
  o Osteoporosis
  o Scoliosis
    ▪ Asymmetric lateral bulge
  o Spondylolisthesis
    ▪ Posterior bulge
  o Ligamentous laxity
- May be a normal variant
  o Typically at L5-S1

Imaging Findings
General Features
- Best imaging clue: Radial outward extension of the anulus fibrosus
CT Findings
- Smooth circumferential apparent enlargement of the disc on axial imaging
- Degenerative changes
  o Anterior and lateral endplate osteophytes
    ▪ May be normal aging
  o Endplate subchondral sclerosis
  o Gas within the disc space
  o Intra-disc calcifications
  o Disc space loss on sagittal reformation

Disc Bulge

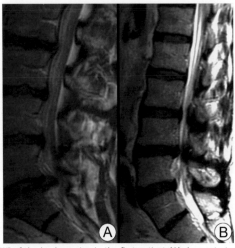

Sagittal T2WI of the lumbar spine in the first patient (A) demonstrates multi-level disc desiccation and disc height loss. Disc bulges are present from L2-3 to L4-5, with disc protrusion at L5-S1. In another patient (B), disc bulges are seen at the same levels. In addition, central stenosis is evident at L2-3 and L3-4.

MR Findings
- Symmetric outward bulging of the disc
- Degenerative changes involving the disc and endplates
  - o Also known as intervertebral osteochondrosis
  - o Diffuse T2 hypointensity within the disc
    - ▪ Initially as linear horizontal hypointensity
    - ▪ Representing fibrosis
    - ▪ Mild hypointensity likely related to normal aging
  - o Disc height loss
  - o Anular tear
  - o Intra-disc gas hypointense on T1WI and T2WI
  - o Fibrovascular marrow in adjacent vertebral bodies
    - ▪ May enhance after intravenous gadolinium
  - o Endplate osteophytes
- Other associated changes
  - o Facet arthropathy
  - o Degenerative spondylolisthesis
  - o Ligamentum flavum hypertrophy
  - o Variable central canal, neural foraminal, and lateral recess narrowing

Discography Findings
- Contrast extension from central site of injection through anular defect
- Provocation of pain suggests symptomatic disk

Differential Diagnosis

Disc Protrusion
- Localized, < 50% of the disc circumference
- Diameter of the herniated disc < diameter at the base

Disc Bulge

Pathology
<u>General</u>
- General Path Comments
  - Whether changes in the intervertebral disc related to normal aging or disc degeneration still controversial
  - May not be able to differentiate on imaging
- Genetics
  - Congenitally weak collagen predisposes to degenerative disc disease
    - Increased incidence of spondylosis in Marfan's syndrome
- Embryology-Anatomy
  - Nucleus pulposus centrally
    - Gelatinous material with high water content and few collagen fibers
  - Anulus fibrosus peripherally
    - Composed of fibrocartilage, with collagen fibers in concentric lamellae
    - Peripheral attachment to the longitudinal ligaments
- Etiology-Pathogenesis
  - With age, water content in nucleus pulposus diminishes
  - Proteoglycans replaced by fibrocartilage and fibrosis
  - Lamellar separation or concentric tear in anulus fibrosus
  - Repetitive micro trauma produces defects in anular attachment at endplate rim
    - Transverse tear
  - Consequent morphologic changes in the disc
  - Disc height loss and bulge also a sequelae of prior discectomy
- Epidemiology
  - High prevalence, > 50% of all asymptomatic adults
    - Increasing with age
    - Increased risk of low back pain, although some are asymptomatic

Clinical Issues
<u>Presentation</u>
- Low back pain - bulge may be incidental and not causative
- Sciatica
- Neurogenic claudication

<u>Natural History</u>
- Symptoms resolve or stabilize with conservative management
- Some develop progressive or chronic neurological deficits and pain

<u>Treatment</u>
- Bed rest
- Analgesic medications
- Surgical decompression in severe spinal stenosis

<u>Prognosis</u>
- Good
- A small percentage may develop multifactorial "failed back syndrome" after surgery

Selected References
1. Consensus statement on nomenclature and classification of lumbar disc pathology by NASS, ASSR, and ASNR. 2001
2. Luoma K et al: Low back pain in relation to lumbar disc degeneration. Spine 25:487-92, 2000
3. Milette PC et al: Differentiating lumbar disc protrusions, disc bulges, and disc with normal contour but abnormal signal intensity. Magnetic resonance imaging with discogenic correlations. Spine 24:44-53, 1999

Anular Tear

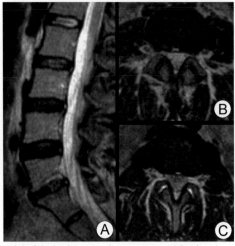

Sagittal T2WI (A) of the lumbar spine demonstrates multilevel anular tears at L3-4, L4-5, and L5-S1. Axial T2WI at L3-4 (B) and L4-5 (C) confirms central anular tears.

Key Facts
- Synonyms: Anular fissure; Anular defect
- Definition: Disruption of concentric collagenous fibers comprising the anulus fibrosus
- Classic imaging appearance
  - Focal high intensity zone in the anulus on T2WI
  - Contrast enhancement on T1WI
- Innervation of the anulus suggests that it may be the source of pain when disrupted
  - Most anular tears are asymptomatic
  - Recurrent meningeal nerve and ventral ramus of somatic spinal nerve are sources of innervation
  - Anular disruption may allow inflammatory substances to leak from nucleus

Imaging Findings
General Features
- Best imaging clue: Abnormal signal focus at the disc margin on MRI
- Typically seen with degenerating disc
MR Findings
- T1WI: Contrast enhancing nidus in disc margin
- T2WI: High signal zone at edge of disc
Other Modality Findings
- Discography demonstrates contrast leak from central site of injection through anulus
- Provocation of pain suggests symptomatic disc
- CECT can show enhancement of disc margin
Imaging Recommendations
- Sagittal heavily T2WI with thin sections
- Contrast-enhanced T1WI

Anular Tear

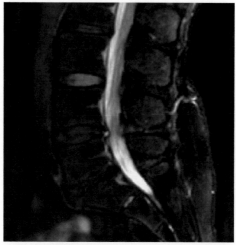

Sagittal T2WI with fat saturation of the lumbar spine in another patient shows an anular tear at L4-5 and disc protrusion at L5-S1.

Differential Diagnosis

Discitis
- Diffuse signal alteration of disc
- Enhancement throughout disc or paralleling endplate(s)
- Abnormal marrow adjacent to interspace
- Epidural abscess may be present

Pathology

General
- Anulus composed of dense, concentric, ordered collagen layers
  - Vertically oriented
  - Attach to hyaline cartilage endplate at rim
  - Contain small blood vessels in outer lateral edge
    - Diminish with age
  - With age, inner anulus expands at expense of nucleus
- Genetics
  - Genetic predisposition to "weak" collagen exists
  - Anular defects associated with certain familial conditions such as Scheuermann's syndrome
- Etiology-Pathogenesis
  - With age, anulus demonstrates focal lamellar thickening
  - Repetitive stress on spinal motion element leads to lamellar separation
    - Concentric tear
  - Micro trauma produces defects in anular attachment at endplate rim
    - Transverse tear
  - Combination of factors including loss of nutrient vessels can lead to lamellar disruption from inner through outer margin
    - Radial fissure or tear
- Epidemiology
  - Autopsy demonstrates high prevalence of tears
    - Increase with age

o Direct association with disc degeneration
o Discography shows presence of anular tears in up to 80% of degenerated discs
o MRI shows anular tears in majority of asymptomatic individuals
   ▪ Some tears seen only on CE T1WI
   ▪ 96% of all tears enhance

Gross Pathologic-Surgical Features
- Separation of lamellar structure in concentric tears
- Transverse disruption of fibers in rim or radial fissures

Microscopic Features
- Granulation tissue with microvascularity invades tears
  o Source of enhancement

Staging or Grading Criteria
- Concentric tears are essentially an aging variant
- Rim tears and radial tears may have clinical consequences in some cases

Clinical Issues

Presentation
- Most tears are incidental findings
- Chronic back pain or sciatica in absence of mechanical nerve root compromise
  o Controversial role of tear
- Discography felt to be provocative test
  o Separates symptomatic tears (internal disc disruption syndrome-IDD) from incidental ones
     ▪ If typical pain reproduced
- No double-blind prospective studies exist to verify IDD theory

Natural History
- Most are asymptomatic or self-limited
  o Scar endpoint of inflammation
- Some felt to be cause of chronic back pain and sciatica

Treatment
- Symptomatic pain relief with NSAIDs
- Chronic pain patients may undergo fusion as last resort

Prognosis
- Good in most symptomatic cases
- Up to 1/3 of chronic pain sufferers have recurrent symptoms despite any therapy

Selected References
1. Saifuddin A et al: The value of lumbar spine magnetic resonance imaging in the demonstration of annular tears. Spine 23(4): 453-7, 1998
2. Stadnik TW et al: Anular tears and disc herniation: prevalence and contrast enhancement on MR images in the absence of low back pain or sciatica. Radiology 206: 49-55, 1998
3. Vernon-Roberts B et al: Pathogenesis of tears of the anulus investigated by multiple-level transaxial analysis of the T12-L1 disc. Spine 22(22): 2641-6, 1997

Disc Herniation

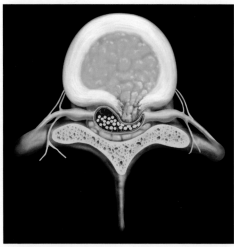

Axial illustration of the lumbar spine depicts a left central anular tear with protruding disc, compressing the thecal sac.

Key Facts
- Synonyms: Herniated nucleus pulposus; Prolapsed disc
- Definition: Localized (< 50% of the disc circumference) displacement of disc material beyond the edges of vertebral ring apophyses
- Classic imaging appearance: Focal disc material extending into spinal canal
- Based on morphology, subdivided into
  - Protrusion
    - Herniated disc with broad base at parent disc, i.e.
    - The greatest diameter of the herniated disc in any plane < the distance between the edges of the base in the same plane
    - Focal: < 25% of the disc circumference
    - Broad-based: > 25%, but < 50% of the disc circumference
  - Extrusion
    - Herniated disc with narrow or no base at parent disc, i.e.,
    - The greatest diameter of the herniated disc in any plane > the distance between the edges of the base in the same plane
    - Sequestered: Extruded disc without continuity to the parent disc
    - Migrated: Disc material displaced away from the site of herniation, regardless of continuity
  - Intravertebral herniation (Schmorl's node)
- Approximately 90% of lumbar disc herniations occur at L4/5 or L5/S1
- In the cervical spine, 60% to 75% occur at C6/7 and 20% to 30% at C5/6

Imaging Findings
General Features
- Best imaging clue: Small mass in spinal canal, contiguous with disc
CT Findings
- Soft tissue disc density extending into spinal canal
  - Displacing nerve root and distorting thecal sac

Disc Herniation

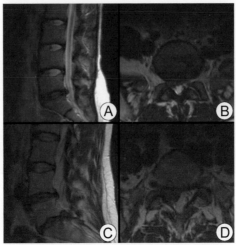

Sagittal and axial T2WI (A, B) demonstrates a central and right subarticular disc protrusion at L5-S1, contacting the traversing right S1 nerve root. In another patient (C, D), there is a right subarticular disc extrusion at L5-S1, distorting the thecal sac and impinging the traversing right S1 nerve root.

MR Findings
- Herniated disc
  - Isointense to parent disc on TWI
  - Iso- to hyperintense on T2WI
    - May be indistinguishable from CSF on T2WI
  - Enhances peripherally after intravenous gadolinium
    - Diffuse enhancement may present on delayed imaging (> 30 minutes after injection)
    - Scar tissue enhances early and homogeneously
  - Sagittal imaging best to discriminate extrusion from protrusion
    - "Mushroom" appearance of disc extrusion due to focal expansion
- Variable extent of nerve impingement and canal stenosis
  - Compressed nerve root may enhance after gadolinium
- Variable degree of degenerative changes in the same or other levels
  - Disc desiccation, bulge +/- anular tear, height loss
  - Schmorl's node (lumbar spine)
  - Endplate changes

Myelography Findings
- Indentation on the anterior thecal sac and the nerve root sleeves

Imaging Recommendations
- If prior surgery, add postgadolinium T1WI in sagittal and axial planes
  - To distinguish postoperative scar from recurrent disc herniation
  - Fat suppression may increase sensitivity

Differential Diagnosis

Peridural Fibrosis
- Early and homogeneous enhancement
- More infiltrative and less masslike
- Surrounds the thecal sac and the nerve root

Disc Herniation

Epidural Hematoma
- More commonly posterior
- More elongated in the cranial-caudal dimension
- Hemorrhagic signal intensity in subacute stage (T1 hyperintensity)

Pathology
General
- General Path Comments
  - o Composed of a combination of nucleus pulposus, fragmented anulus, cartilage, and fragmented apophyseal bone
- Genetics
  - o Congenitally weak collagen predisposes to degenerative disc disease
    - Increased incidence of spondylosis in Marfan's syndrome
- Embryology-Anatomy
  - o Nucleus pulposus centrally
    - Gelatinous material with high water content and few collagen fibers
    - Water content diminishes with age, replaced by fibrocartilage
  - o Anulus fibrosus peripherally
    - Composed of fibrocartilage, with collagen fibers in concentric lamellae
    - Peripheral attachment to the longitudinal ligaments (anuloligamentous complex)
- Etiology-Pathogenesis
  - o Degenerative or posttraumatic breach in the anulus
  - o Disc material extends through the defect
  - o Protrusions may be contained by thinned anuloligamentous complex
- Epidemiology
  - o Up to one-third of asymptomatic adults have one or more lumbar disc herniations by age 60
  - o Affects all age groups and ethnicities

Clinical Issues
Presentation
- Neck/low back pain (may be incidental), sciatica, radiculopathy
Natural History
- Symptoms resolve or stabilize with conservative management
- Some develop progressive or chronic neurological deficits and pain
Treatment
- Bed rest and analgesic medications
  - o No or minimal neurological impairment
- Discectomy if conservative treatment fails or neurological deficits present
Prognosis
- Good
- A small percentage may develop multi-factorial "failed back syndrome" after surgery

Selected References
1. Consensus statement on nomenclature and classification of lumbar disc pathology by NASS, ASSR, and ASNR. 2001
2. Moore RJ et al: The origin and fate of herniated lumbar intervertebral disc tissue. Spine 21: 2149-55, 1996
3. Hueftle MG et al: Lumbar spine: postoperative MR imaging with Gd-DTPA. Radiology 167: 817-24, 1988

Disc Extrusion

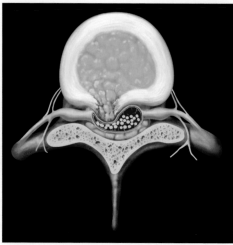

Focal disc herniation. Drawing depicts anulus fibrosus disruption leading to a right paracentral focal disc herniation. The extruded disc contents produce ventral thecal sac compression and narrowing of the lateral recess.

Key Facts
- Synonym(s): Extruded disc, focal disc herniation with extrusion
- Definition: Herniation is defined as disc material outside the confines of the disc space
  - Additional criteria for disc extrusion requires that the diameter of extruded fragment is greater than that of the fragment neck at parent disc space
- Classic imaging appearance: Focal "mushroom" configuration of herniated disc material
- New NASS/ASNR consensus statement for lumbar disc terminology
  - No consensus statement available for cervical or thoracic discs, but similar terminology is in common usage

Imaging Findings
General Features
- Best imaging clue: Peripheral disc margins "mushroom" larger than base in at least one plane
CT Findings
- Soft-tissue mass protruding from disc space into spinal canal
  - Effaces epidural fat and compresses thecal sac
- Difficult to discriminate protrusion from extrusion in axial plane
MR Findings
- Disc fragment is frequently hyperintense relative to native disc material
- Disc material "mushrooms" out after leaving confines of disc space
- Extrusion characteristics are usually most obvious in the sagittal plane
- Extruded disc material enhances peripherally in subacute phase
  - Permits distinction from vascular scar tissue which enhances homogeneously

Disc Extrusion

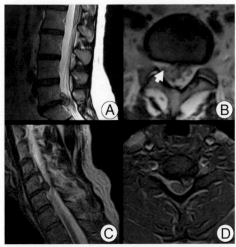

Lumbar spine: Sagittal (A) and axial T2WI (B) show large L5/S1 parasagittal extruded disc herniation with displacement of the transiting right S1 nerve root (arrow). Cervical spine. (C, D) Large paracentral disc herniation "tents" the PLL and compresses the left ventral lateral spinal cord.

Other Modality Findings
- Myelography
  - Soft-tissue density material compresses the anterior thecal sac and nerve root sleeves

Imaging Recommendations
- T1WI and T2WI in sagittal and axial planes
- Contrast administration in postoperative patients to distinguish scar from recurrent disc herniation

Differential Diagnosis

Disc Protrusion
- Greatest distance in any plane between disc material edges beyond the disc space is less than the distance between the edges at the base
- The height of the base cannot exceed the height of the intervertebral space in the sagittal plane

Post-operative Scar Tissue
- Mass effect; frequently encircles nerve root
- Enhances avidly for several years following surgery; recurrent disc herniation usually does not

Nerve Sheath Tumor
- Neurofibroma or Schwannoma
- Avid contrast enhancement
- May show characteristic "dumbbell" configuration

Epidural Hematoma
- Characteristic blood signal in subacute stage; acute stage may mimic extrusion

Disc Extrusion

Pathology

<u>General</u>
- General Path Comments
  - o Extruded material can be cartilage, fragmented apophyseal bone, fragmented anulus, or nucleus pulposus
- Etiology-Pathogenesis
  - o By definition requires a breach of the anulus; protrusions may only thin and distend the anulus
    - ▪ Disc material herniates through the anular defect, either in the midline or paracentral (just lateral to the PLL margin)
    - ▪ "Expansion" of extruded disc material after passing through the relatively narrow anular disruption produces the characteristic "mushroom" appearance
- Epidemiology
  - o Herniations are common
    - ▪ Up to one-third of asymptomatic adults have one or more lumbar herniations by age 60
    - ▪ Affect all age groups and ethnicities

<u>Gross Pathologic-Surgical Features</u>
- Location of disc herniations
  - o Approximately 90% of lumbar disc herniations occur at L4/5 or L5/S1
  - o In the cervical spine, 60 to 75% occur at C6/7 and 20 to 30% at C5/6
- Additional important terms with surgical planning implications
  - o An extrusion is called a sequestration if the displaced disc material has completely lost continuity with the parent disc
  - o The term migration implies displacement of disc material away from the site of extrusion, regardless of whether it is sequestrated or not
  - o Posteriorly displaced disc material is often constrained by the posterior anuloligamentous complex

Clinical Issues

<u>Presentation</u>
- Back/neck pain, with or without extremity pain
- Loss of relevant deep tendon reflexes in dermatomal distribution of affected root(s)
- Myelopathy from significant cord compression (cervical, thoracic)

<u>Natural History</u>
- Many patients improve with conservative management only
- Others develop progressive or chronic neurological deficits and pain

<u>Treatment</u>
- First line is conservative nonoperative management
  - o Reasonable approach if no neurological deficits and pain is manageable
- Surgical discectomy if conservative treatment fails or neurological deficits

Selected References
1. Millette PC et al: Reporting lumbar disk abnormalities: At last, consensus! AJNR 22(3): 428-30, 2001
2. Beattie PF et al: Associations between patient report of symptoms and anatomic impairment visible on lumbar magnetic resonance imaging. Spine 25(7): 819-28, 2000
3. Moore RJ et al: The origin and fate of herniated lumbar intervertebral disc tissue. Spine 21(18): 2149-55, 1996

Facet Arthropathy

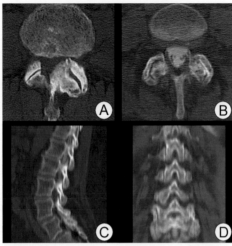

(A) Axial CT shows severe left unilateral facet overgrowth. (B) Axial CT myelogram (different patient) shows bilateral facet overgrowth with articular joint space loss. (C, D) Sagittal and coronal reformatted post myelogram images show severe facet degenerative changes at L4/5, L5/S1 (compare to normal T12/L1 level).

Key Facts
- Synonym(s): Facet arthrosis, degenerative facet disease, degenerative joint disease
- Definition: Osteoarthritis of the synovially-lined apophyseal joints
- Classic imaging appearance: Osseous facet overgrowth impinging on the neural foramina; articular joint space narrowing
- Facet joint degeneration begins in first two decades of life
  - Identifiable to varying degrees in majority of adults
  - Virtually universal after age 60 years
- Associated with synovial cysts, degenerative disc disease

Imaging Findings
General Features
- Best imaging clue: Osseous facet overgrowth and cartilage erosion with joint space narrowing; frequently seen in conjunction with spondylosis
CT Findings
- Facet joint osteophytes producing foraminal narrowing
- "Mushroom cap" facet appearance
- Joint space narrowing with sclerosis and bone eburnation
- Intra-articular gas ("vacuum phenomenon")
MR Findings
- Osteophyte proliferation limiting neural foramina
- Joint space narrowing, thinning of articular cartilage
- Conversely, some patients show variable synovial thickening
  - Irritation of the synovium can produce synovial hyperplasia with paradoxical joint space widening
  - Frequently see motion at affected levels on dynamic upright flexion-extension plain films
Other Modality Findings
- Plain films demonstrate facet arthrosis well, not soft tissues

Facet Arthropathy

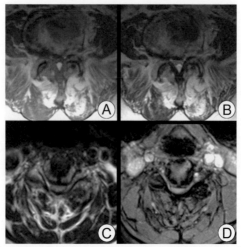

Lumbar spine: (A, B) Axial T1WI, T2WI show facet overgrowth, prominent ligamentum flavum, and asymmetric synovial space loss (left > right). Cervical spine: (C, D) Axial T2WI, GRE images show left facet complex enlargement with joint space narrowing and hypointense signal (sclerosis).

- CT myelography elegantly portrays facet relationship to adjacent contrast-opacified thecal sac and nerve root sleeves

Imaging Recommendations
- Plain films useful to demonstrate presence and severity of facet degenerative changes
- Sagittal and axial T1WI and T2WI best demonstrate degenerative facet compression of adjacent thecal sac and fat-filled neural foramina
- Consider CT myelography if MRI contraindications or when MRI does not adequately demonstrate facet relationship to neural foramina

Differential Diagnosis

Healing Facet Fracture
- Attempt to elicit trauma history and search for fracture line

Inflammatory Arthritides
- Look for ankylosis or erosions
- Search for associated disease findings in other characteristic locations
  - SI joint erosions or ankylosis (ankylosing spondylitis, psoriatic arthritis, Reiter's disease)
  - Cranial settling, atlanto-axial subluxation (rheumatoid arthritis)

Pathology

General
- General Path Comments
  - Degenerative (hypertrophic) inflammatory changes in synovial joints
  - Normal bone mineralization (in contrast to rheumatoid arthritis)
  - Joint traction during subluxation may produce gas in joint ("vacuum phenomenon")
- Etiology-Pathogenesis
  - Frequently seen in aging population

Facet Arthropathy

- o May see earlier presentation after trauma, with kyphosis/scoliosis, or following surgical fusion at adjacent level

Gross Pathologic-Surgical Features

- Most common locations
  - o Mid/lower cervical spine, lower lumbar spine
  - o Thoracic spine uncommon
- Joint space narrowing, capsular laxity may permit subluxation of the superior facet on the inferior facet (degenerative spondylolisthesis)

Microscopic Features

- Findings are similar to those seen in synovial joints at other locations
  - o Osseous proliferation
  - o Preservation of bone density
  - o Fibrillation and erosion of articular joint cartilage

Clinical Issues

Presentation

- Mechanical pain, radiculopathy, myelopathy (rarely), and/or spondylolisthesis
- May be incidental and asymptomatic

Natural History

- Can show progressive symptoms/signs

Treatment

- Mechanical pain – conservative medical therapy
- Foraminal narrowing with radiculopathy – foraminotomy
- Subluxation
  - o Cervical – transarticular fusion with lateral mass screws or anterior cervical discectomy and fusion
  - o Lumbar – Posterior fusion with pedicle screws and rods (rarely in conjunction with anterior interbody fusion)

Prognosis

- Variable (depending on severity)

Selected References
1. Grob D: Surgery in the degenerative cervical spine. Spine 23(24): 2674-83, 1998
2. Mehta M et al: Mechanical back pain and the facet joint syndrome. Disabil Rehabil 16(1): 2-12, 1994
3. Oegema TR Jr et al: The inter-relationship of facet joint osteoarthritis and degenerative disc disease. Br J Rheumatol 30(Suppl 1): 16-20, 1991

Facet Joint Synovial Cyst

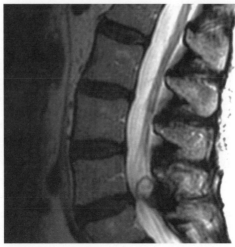

Sagittal T2WI reveals a hyperintense lesion with a thin hypointense rim located posterolaterally in the spinal canal at the L4-5 level.

Key Facts
- Contiguous with degenerated facet joints
- May be filled with synovial or hemorrhagic fluid
- Thickened synovium
- Possible bone erosion

Imaging Findings
<u>General Features</u>
- Best imaging clue: Posterolateral extradural cystic lesion abutting the facet joint at L4-5

<u>CT Findings</u>
- Difficult to detect because of fluid density
- Made more visible by hemorrhage and mural calcifications

<u>MR Findings</u>
- Variable, signal intensity because of serous, proteinaceous, or hemorrhagic contents
- Enhancing wall after IV gadolinium administration
- Degenerative changes in the parent and the contralateral facet joints

<u>Conventional Myelography Findings</u>
- Nonspecific posterolateral extradural mass

Differential Diagnosis
<u>Extruded Disc Fragment</u>
- More lobulated compared to the more spherical cyst
- Not contiguous with the facet joint
- Rarely posterolateral

<u>Ganglion Cyst</u>
- Difficult to distinguish by imaging
- Contains myxoid material
- Lined by fibrous connective tissue capsule

Facet Joint Synovial Cyst

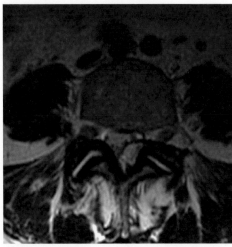

Axial T2WI shows the hyperintense lesion contiguous with the left L4-5 facet joint, distorting the thecal sac and narrowing the left subarticular recess.

Pathology
General
- General Path Comments
  o Thickened connective tissue and synovium
  o Invariably associated with degenerated disc and facet disease
- Etiology-Pathogenesis
  o Stress loading on the lumbar spine
  o Facet osteoarthropathy
  o Joint fluid accumulation
  o Synovial proliferation
- Epidemiology
  o More commonly in females
  o Fifth and sixth decades

Microscopic Features
- Serous, proteinaceous and or hemorrhagic material
- Lined with hypervascular synovium

Clinical Issues
Presentation
- Principal presenting symptom: Low back pain
- Acute pain from hemorrhage
- Symptoms related to spinal stenosis

Treatment
- Laminectomy with excision of the cyst
- Less permanent
  o Percutaneous cyst puncture and drainage
  o Steroid injection

Prognosis
- High success rate in symptomatic patients

Facet Joint Synovial Cyst

Selected References
1. Jackson DE et al: Intraspinal Synovial Cysts: MR Imaging. Radiology 170 (2): 527-30, 1989
2. Liu SS et al: Synovial Cysts of the Lumbosacral Spine: Diagnosis by MR Imaging. AJNR 10 November/December: 1239-42, 1989

Spondylolysis with Spondylolisthesis

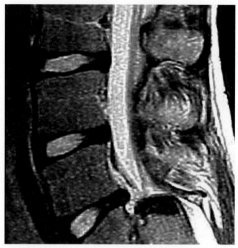

Sagittal T2WI image reveals grade 4 anterolisthesis of L5 on S1.

Key Facts
- Definition: Defects in the pars interarticularis thought to result from repetitive stress injury
- Classic imaging appearance: Discontinuity in the neck of the "Scotty dog" on oblique views of the lumbar spine
- Other key facts
  - Often associated with spondylolisthesis
  - 10-15% unilateral defects
    - Unilateral healing or union of a defect that was initially bilateral

Imaging Findings
General Features
- Best imaging clue: Elongation of the spinal canal at the level of the pars defects on axial MR imaging
Plain Film Findings
- Break in the neck of the "Scotty dog" as the pars interarticularis defect on oblique views of the standing lumbar spine
CT Findings
- "Incomplete ring" sign on axial imaging
  - May simulate "extra" facet joints
- Spondylolisthesis and foraminal narrowing on sagittal reformatted images
MR Findings
- Focally decreased signal in the pars on sagittal and axial T1 and T2 weighted sequences
- Elongation of the spinal canal at the level of the pars defects
- More horizontal configuration of the affected neural foramina on sagittal imaging
- Loss of fat surrounding the exiting nerve roots

Differential Diagnosis: Mimickers of Spondylolysis on Sagittal MR
Sclerosis of the Neck of the Pars
- May represent "healed" pars lysis

Spondylolysis with Spondylolisthesis

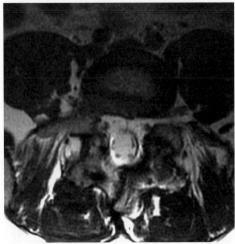

Axial T2WI through L5-S1 in a second patient shows elongated AP dimension of the spinal canal at this level. Bilateral L5 pars defects are evident.

Partial Volume Imaging of the Spur Arising From the Superior Facet Slightly Lateral to the Pars
Partial Facetectomy
Blastic Metastasis Replacing the Marrow of the Pars

Pathology
General
- Genetics
  - Predisposing familial conditions to spondylolysis
    - Marfan's syndrome
    - Osteogenesis imperfecta
    - Osteopetrosis
    - Inherited traits
- Etiology-Pathogenesis
  - Repetitive exposure to simultaneous forces of muscle contraction, gravity, and rotational force
  - Participation in gymnastics, weight lifting, wrestling, and football at a young age
  - Repeated micro-fractures of the pars interarticularis
- Epidemiology
  - 4.4% at age 6
  - 6% in adults
  - Prevalence of 5-7% in the general population
  - 2 to 3:1 male to female ratio

Clinical Issues
Presentation
- Asymptomatic in young children
- Chronic low back pain in older children and adults
- Exacerbated by rigorous activities

Spondylolysis with Spondylolisthesis

- Radiculopathy and cauda equina syndrome in spondylolysis with high-grade spondylolisthesis

Natural History
- Little progression with horizontal sacrum
  - Lumbosacral angle > or = 100 degrees
- Disease progression with vertical sacrum
  - Lumbosacral angle < 100 degrees
- Progression from grade 1 spondylolisthesis
  - Superior vertebral body subluxed by one-fourth of a vertebral body
- To grade 2
  - Subluxation by half a vertebral body
- To grade 3
  - Subluxation by three-fourths of a vertebral body
- To grade 4
  - Subluxation by the whole width of a vertebral body

Treatment
- Conservative measures in patients with grade 1 and 2 spondylolisthesis
  - Back brace treatment
  - Modification of activity
- Surgical interventions in symptomatic patients with any degree of spondylolisthesis
  - Gradual traction in hyperextension
  - Cast immobilization
  - Posterolateral fusion

Prognosis
- Conservative measures in patients with < 50% slips
  - Two-thirds success rate of symptomatic relief
- Posterolateral fusion in patients with > 50% slips
  - 60 to 70% solid fusion rate
  - 10 to 12% complication rate of neurological deficit following fusion

Selected References
1. Ulmer J et al: MR Imaging of Lumbar Spondylolysis: The Importance of Ancillary Observations. AJR 169:233-9, 1997
2. Reynolds R: Spondylolysis and Spondylolisthesis. Seminars in Spine Surgery 4:235-47, 1992
3. Johnson D et al: MR Imaging of the Pars Interarticularis. AJR 152:327-32, 1989

Ligamentous Ossifications

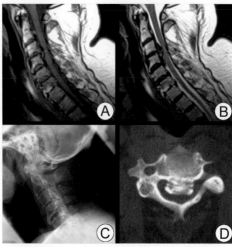

(A, B) Sagittal T1-, T2WIs show ossification of the posterior longitudinal ligament (OPLL) producing cord compression. Note marrow signal in prominent OPLL. (C) Lateral plain film shows same finding (more subtle). (D) Axial CT confirms OPLL.

Key Facts
- Synonym(s): Diffuse idiopathic skeletal hyperostosis (DISH), ossification of the posterior longitudinal ligament (OPLL, "Japanese disease"), ossification of the ligamentum flavum (OLF)
- Definition: Ossification of spinal ligament(s); appearance and clinical manifestations depend on which ligament is abnormal
- Classic imaging appearance: Thickening of ligamentous structure, ossification on CT, and either hypointense or hyperintense MRI appearance depending on amount and composition of marrow elements.
- Can involve any spinal ligament, but most important are
  - Anterior longitudinal ligament (ALL) – DISH
  - Posterior longitudinal ligament (PLL) – OPLL
  - Ligamentum flavum (LF) – OLF

Imaging Findings
General Features
- OPLL is most common in the cervical, thoracic spine
- DISH presents first in the thoracic spine; later in cervical, lumbar spine
- OLF is most common in the mid-cervical, lower thoracic spine
- Best imaging clues: Flowing multilevel ossification anterior (DISH) or posterior (OPLL) to the vertebral bodies, relatively minimal degenerative disc disease, and absent facet ankylosis
CT Findings
- DISH – Three strict diagnostic criteria
  - Flowing ossification along at least 4 contiguous vertebral bodies
  - No apophyseal or SI joint ankylosis
  - Relatively minimal degenerative disc changes
- OPLL
  - PLL ossification narrows AP spinal canal
  - Characteristic "upside down T" configuration on axial images

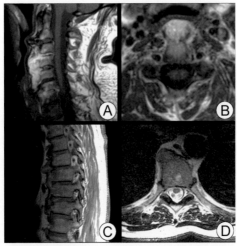

(A, B) Sagittal and Axial T1WI show exuberant DISH displacing aerodigestive tract anteriorly. Marrow signal is predominantly fatty. (C) Sagittal T1WI (different patient) showing classic thoracic DISH over four contiguous bodies. (D) Axial T2WI depicts characteristic involvement of ALL on side opposite to aorta.

- OLF
  - o Calcification or bone deposition in the ligamentum flavum

MR Findings
- DISH
  - o Diagnostic criteria same as CT
  - o May be hypointense if predominantly calcified, or isointense to hyperintense if marrow fat present
- OPLL
  - o Characteristic "upside-down T" configuration on axial images
  - o Posterior flowing ossification over multiple levels on sagittal images
  - o Usually low signal intensity on all pulse sequences
    - ▪ High signal if marrow fat
- OLF – signal characteristics similar to DISH

Other Modality Findings
- Plain films
  - o Shows flowing anterior (DISH) or posterior (OPLL) osteophytes well
  - o Cannot assess spinal cord status

Imaging Recommendations
- Sagittal T1WI, T2WI to evaluate spinal cord, ligamentous ossification
- Axial T2WI or T1WI images to evaluate stenosis degree
- GRE may exaggerate stenosis due to magnetic susceptibility effects
- CT imaging (if necessary) to confirm MR diagnosis

Differential Diagnosis

Spondylosis
- Rarely contiguous across four or more vertebral levels
- Confined to vicinity of interspace
- More substantial facet and disc degenerative changes than DISH, OPLL
- Absence of characteristic "T- shaped" OPLL configuration

Ligamentous Ossifications

Meningioma or Calcified Herniated Disc
- Meningiomas almost always enhance; look for dural tail, smooth margins
- Lacks characteristic multilevel "T" shape of OPLL

Pathology
General
- General Path Comments
  - DISH, OPLL frequently co-exist; OLF uncommon
- Etiology-Pathogenesis
  - DISH – exaggerated response to new bone formation stimuli
  - OPLL – unknown; but postulated etiologies include infectious agents, autoimmune disorders, trauma, and diabetes mellitus
- Epidemiology
  - DISH
    - Men > women (2:1); middle age and older adults
    - Association with diabetes, alcohol intake, and poor dietary intake of calcium, carotene, vitamins A,C, E
  - OPLL
    - 2% prevalence in Japan; sporadic cases worldwide
    - Men > women (2:1); most commonly diagnosed age 50 - 60 years

Gross Pathologic-Surgical Features
- DISH does not produce spinal stenosis by definition
  - Anterior osteophytes may displace esophagus and cause dysphagia or reduce spine mobility
  - Curious predisposition to right anterior thoracic spine
- OPLL produces symptomatic myelopathy when canal diameter reduced
  - Most common in the midcervical (C3-C5), midthoracic (T4-T7) spine
  - Myelopathy almost universal if canal < 6mm; rare if > 14mm

Clinical Issues
Presentation
- DISH – incidental finding, spinal stiffness, or dysphagia
- OPLL – incidental finding or myelopathy referable to stenosis level
- OLF – generally incidental observation; may produce dorsal thoracic spinal cord compression

Treatment
- DISH – osteophyte resection if symptomatic
- OPLL, OLF – posterior decompression (laminectomy or laminoplasty)

Prognosis
- DISH is usually incidental finding without additive morbidity or mortality
- 22% of OPLL develop progressive spastic paresis progressing to paralysis

Selected References
1. Matsunaga S et al: Pathogenesis of myelopathy in patients with ossification of the posterior longitudinal ligament. J Neurosurg (Spine 2) 96: 168-172, 2002
2. Sakou T et al: Recent progress in the study of pathogenesis of ossification of the posterior longitudinal ligament. J Orthop Sci 5(3): 310-5, 2000
3. Ehara S et al: Paravertebral ligamentous ossification: DISH, OPLL and OLF. Eur J Radiol 27(3): 196-205, 1998

Acquired Spinal Stenosis

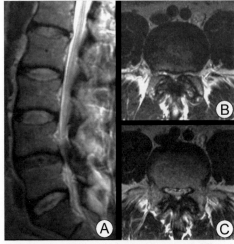

Acquired spinal stenosis. Sagittal T2WI (A) demonstrates diffuse lumbar canal narrowing, most severe at L4-5. Axial T2WI (B) confirms spinal stenosis secondary to disc bulge, ligamentum flavum laxity, hypertrophied facets. (C) Congenitally short pedicles with narrowed lateral recesses are present.

Key Facts
- Synonym: Spondylosis
- Definition
  - Spinal canal and neural foraminal narrowing in the cervical spine
  - Additional lateral recess narrowing in the lumber spine
  - Secondary to multifactorial degenerative changes
- Classic imaging appearance
  - Completely effaced subarachnoid space at the disc levels in the cervical spine – "washboard spine"
  - Trefoil appearance of the lumbar spinal canal on axial imaging
  - Obliterated perineural fat in the lumbar neural foramina on sagittal imaging
  - Narrowed lumbar lateral recess on axial imaging
- Other key facts
  - Congenitally short pedicles often contribute to acquired spinal stenosis
  - The degree of spinal stenosis may not correlate with symptomatology
  - Most common in the lower cervical and lumber spine where there is most mobility
  - MRI equivalent to CT myelogram in diagnosing lumbar spinal stenosis, but provides additional information on the spinal cord
  - MRI of the cervical spine may overestimate neural foraminal stenosis

Imaging Findings
General Features
- Best imaging clue
  - Completely effaced cerebral spinal fluid in the cervical spine at the disc levels
  - Sagittal diameter of the lumbar canal less than 1.2 cm
CT Myelogram Findings
- Central canal and neural foraminal narrowing in the cervical spine

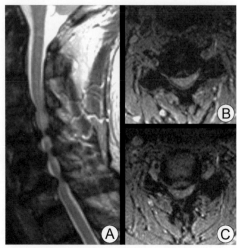

Sagittal T2WI (A) demonstrates multi-level stenosis from C3-4 to C6-7 due to disc-osteophyte complexes. The cord is atrophied with vague T2 hyperintensity at the level of C4. In addition, axial GRE images (B, C) show bilateral neural foraminal narrowing secondary to uncovertebral and facet hypertrophy.

- Additional lateral recess narrowing in the lumbar spine
- Variable degree of cord and nerve root impingement

MR Findings
- Lumbar spine
  - Hourglass appearance of the central canal on sagittal T2WI
  - Obliterated perineural fat in the neural foramina on sagittal imaging
  - Degenerative disc disease with variable degree of herniation
  - Vertebral endplate osteophytes
  - Elongated and redundant nerve roots above and below the level of stenosis
  - Trefoil appearance of the spinal canal on axial imaging
  - Narrowed lateral recess on axial imaging
  - Thickened ligamentum flavum
  - Facet joint hypertrophy
  - Enhancing and crowded nerve roots
  - Short pedicles
- Cervical spine
  - Disc-osteophyte complex protruding into the canal
  - Obliterated subarachnoid space at the disc levels
  - Variable degree of cord compression
  - Intramedullary T2 hyperintensity representing myelomalacia, demyelination, or edema
    - May enhance after gadolinium
  - Uncovertebral and facet joint hypertrophy
  - Narrowing of the neural foramina

Differential Diagnosis
Ossification of the Posterior Longitudinal Ligament
- A cause of cervical spinal stenosis

Acquired Spinal Stenosis

- Thick band of hypointensity along the posterior vertebral margin
- Central hyperintensity within the band represents fatty marrow

Epidural Hemorrhage
- Variable signal intensity depending on the evolving hemoglobin
- Acute onset of symptoms

Pathology
General
- General Path Comments
  - Age related degenerative disease
- Etiology-Pathogenesis
  - Degenerative changes involving the discs, vertebral endplates, uncovertebral joints (cervical spine), facet joints, and ligamentum flavum
  - Congenitally short pedicles often present
- Epidemiology
  - Fifth decade and later, more commonly in men

Clinical Issues
Presentation
- Lumbar stenosis
  - Chronic low back pain
  - Bilateral lower extremity pain, paresthesia, and weakness
  - Exacerbated by prolonged standing and walking
  - Relieved by squatting or sitting (flexion)
- Cervical spondylosis
  - Chronic neck pain radiating to the occiput and upper extremities
  - Upper extremity numbness
  - Spastic paraparesis
  - Loss of position and vibration sense

Natural History
- Progressive neurologic deficits

Treatment
- Lumber spine
  - Analgesic medications
  - Surgical decompression with laminectomies and fusion
- Cervical spine
  - Analgesic medications
  - Soft collar immobilization and traction
  - Depending on the site of compression
    - Anterior corpectomy or inner-body arthrodesis
    - Posterior decompression with laminectomies or open-door laminaplasties with or without foraminotomies

Prognosis
- Favorable outcome if treated early
- The severity and duration of preoperative neurologic deficits predictive of the degree of neurologic recovery

Selected References
1. Alfieri KM et al: MR imaging of spinal stenosis. Applied Radiology. August:18-26, 1997
2. Amunosen T et al: Lumbar spinal stenosis: clinical and radiologic features. Spine 20:1178-86, 1995
3. Modic MT et al: Imaging of degenerative disease of the cervical spine. Clin Orthop 239:109-20, 1989

Rheumatoid Arthritis

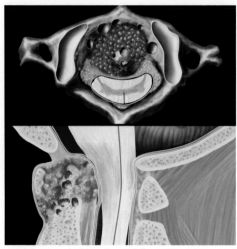

Axial and sagittal drawings depict exuberant inflammatory pannus eroding the dens and adjacent atlas, resulting in forward translation of C1 relative to C2, central canal narrowing, and cord compression.

Key Facts
- Synonym: RA
- Definition: Inflammatory arthritis of unknown etiology producing osteopenia, erosions, but minimal productive change
- Classic imaging appearance: Osteopenic patient with C1/2 subluxation and dens erosion
- Symmetric arthritis primarily affects appendicular skeleton
- Tendency to spare the axial skeleton
  - Exception is the cervical spine, where it is clinically important
- Primary manifestations found in hands, feet, knees, hips, cervical spine, shoulder, and elbow (in decreasing frequency)

Imaging Findings
General Features
- Best imaging clue: Osteopenic patient with C1/2 subluxation
- Characteristic imaging features
  - Widened atlanto-dentate interval (between anterior C1 ring and dens)
  - Odontoid erosions
  - Atlanto-axial impaction (may be occult)
  - Apophyseal joint erosions (rarely ankylosis)
    - Ankylosis is common in Juvenile Chronic Arthritis (JCA)
  - Mechanical spinous process erosion
- Disc and adjacent vertebral body destruction (rare)
  - Synovitis extending from joint of Luschka
  - Difficult to distinguish from infection – may require biopsy
CT Findings
- Demonstrates osteopenia and erosions well
- Look for C1/2 subluxation

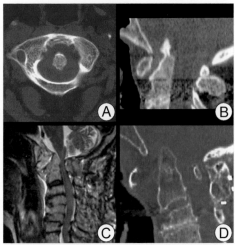

Axial CT (A) shows C1/2 subluxation. Sagittal CT reformat (B) (different patient) demonstrates marked cranial settling and, dens erosions. Sagittal T2WI (C) and sagittal CT reformat (D) reveals marked C1/2 subluxation and cranial settling producing cord compression.

MR Findings
- Best for demonstrating soft-tissue pannus, odontoid erosions, and presence/degree of cord compression
- Dynamic changes from atlanto-axial subluxation and cranial settling can be assessed in flexion and extension

Other Modality Findings
- Plain films evaluate cervical spine and appendicular skeleton well
  - Important for making initial diagnosis
  - Upright flexion-extension films show presence/degree of instability
    - 33% of RA patients exhibit C1/2 instability on flexion
  - Instability at C1/2 may be missed in neutral position

Imaging Recommendations
- Evaluate craniovertebral junction in RA patients carefully
- Plain cervical films in flexion/extension to assess for C1/2 instability
- Plain films of hands and/or feet to confirm diagnosis
- Thin section bone algorithm CT with sagittal and coronal reformats to assess bone density, plan screw placement for fusion
- MR imaging with sagittal and axial thin sections to evaluate for cranial settling, cord compression, subluxation

Differential Diagnosis

Seronegative Spondyloarthropathy
- Psoriatic arthritis, Reiter's disease, ankylosing spondylitis
- Productive changes, relatively preserved bone density, and characteristic SI joint involvement distinguish from RA

Cervical Trauma
- Traumatic disruption of transverse ligament can produce C1/2 instability
- Subacute dens fracture can simulate RA at C1/2 but lacks other RA signs

- Search for trauma history, bone marrow edema and associated fractures, ligamentous edema from injury

Pathology
<u>General</u>
- General Path Comments
  - o RF factor may be negative initially
    - ▪ Eventually positive in up to 95% of RA patients
  - o Polyarticular synovial inflammation and articular destruction
- Etiology-Pathogenesis
  - o Common arthritis of unknown etiology
- Epidemiology
  - o Young to middle-aged patients
  - o Female-to-male ratio 2–3:1
  - o Cervical spine is involved in approximately 50% of afflicted patients
    - ▪ Thoracic and lumbar spine are rarely involved significantly

<u>Gross Pathologic-Surgical Features</u>
- Atlanto-axial findings are most common manifestation of cervical spine RA
  - o Laxity of transverse ligament permits subluxation of the anterior C1 ring relative to the dens
  - o Pannus can cause cord compression

Clinical Issues
<u>Presentation</u>
- Chronic or episodic symptoms
  - o Early morning stiffness
  - o Pain
  - o Tendon contractures and ruptures
  - o ESR elevation paralleling disease activity
  - o Cervical myelopathy
    - ▪ Only a small proportion develop clinically apparent myelopathy

<u>Treatment</u>
- C1/2 transarticular surgical fusion for atlanto-axial subluxation
- Transoral odontoid resection for dens/pannus cord compression

Selected References
1. Reijnierse M et al: Neurologic dysfunction in patients with rheumatoid arthritis of the cervical spine. Predictive value of clinical, radiographic and MR imaging parameters. Eur Radiol 11(3): 467-73, 2001
2. Neva MH et al: Prevalence of radiological changes in the cervical spine-a cross sectional study after 20 years from presentation of rheumatoid arthritis. J Rheumatol 27(1): 90-3, 2000
3. Yoshida K T et al: Progression of rheumatoid arthritis of the cervical spine: radiographic and clinical evaluation. J Orthop Sci 4(6): 399-406, 1999

Seronegative Spondyloarthropathy

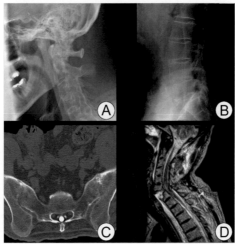

Ankylosing spondylitis. (A) Lateral plain film of cervical spine shows "bamboo spine." (B) Lateral lumbar plain film shows syndesmophytes and squared corners. (C) Axial CT reveals SI joint ankylosis. (D) Sagittal T2WI demonstrates typical AS fracture pattern with pseudoarthrosis, and cord contusion.

Key Facts
- Definition: RF (rheumatoid factor) negative inflammatory arthritis
- Classic imaging appearance: Sacroiliitis, productive osseous changes of axial skeleton, and mixed productive/erosive arthritis of proximal joints
- Ankylosing spondylitis (AS), reactive arthritis (formerly called Reiter's disease), psoriatic arthritis
- Afflicted patients are frequently HLA – B27 haplotype positive
  - 95% AS, 80% Reiter's, 50% psoriatic patients are positive
  - 6-8% of normal population is HLA – B27 positive

Imaging Findings
General Features
- Best imaging clue: SI joint erosion or ankylosis
- In some cases may be able to specifically diagnose arthritis type
  - Ankylosing spondylitis
    - Delicate contiguous thoracolumbar syndesmophytes ("bamboo spine"), generally symmetric SI joint disease
  - Reactive arthritis and psoriatic arthritis
    - Bulky asymmetric lateral osteophytes, with skip segments interspersed, and asymmetric SI joint disease (especially in early disease)

CT Findings
- Normal bone density (distinguishes from RA)
- Thoracic kyphosis, SI joint erosion (early) or ankylosis (late), enthesopathy
- Fusion across disc spaces, syndesmophytes and squared vertebral bodies (AS) or bulky lateral osteophytes (reactive and psoriatic arthritides)

MR Findings
- Thoracic kyphosis, straightening of lumbar and cervical spine

Seronegative Spondyloarthropathy

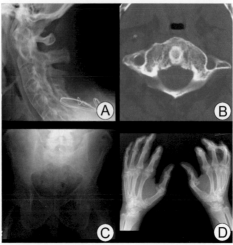

Psoriatic arthritis. (A) Lateral plain film shows extensive cervical ankylosis; posterior fusion is for prior injury. (B) Axial CT shows complete fusion at C1/2. (C) AP plain film shows SI joint ankylosis and abnormal pelvic tilt from lumbar ankylosis. (D) PA plain film of hands shows psoriatic arthritis changes.

- Syndesmophytes and squared vertebral bodies (AS) or bulky lateral osteophytes (reactive and psoriatic arthritides)
- Marrow in disc spaces (later stages), preservation of central canal

Other Modality Findings
- Plain films excellent modality for initial diagnosis
- Show syndesmophytes, SI joint, and extremity changes well

Imaging Recommendations
- Start with plain films; use CT if plain films are negative
- MR/CT in combination to evaluate bone and cord status following trauma

Differential Diagnosis

Rheumatoid Arthritis
- Combination of productive and erosive disease help distinguish seronegative spondyloarthropathy from RA
- Late AS may show osteopenia, but ankylosis will distinguish the two

Pathology

General
- RF negative, elevated ESR
  - AS
    - Axial skeleton and proximal large joints
    - ALL/PLL/ anulus fibrosus ossification produces syndesmophytes
  - Reactive Arthritis
    - Bulky asymmetric lateral thoracolumbar osteophytes (calcifications of periarticular soft tissues that become contiguous with spine) with skip segments
    - Erosive arthropathy with periostitis usually seen first in feet
    - Bilateral sacroiliitis less common than AS (30%); asymmetric early, symmetric late

- o Psoriatic arthritis
    - Spine findings indistinguishable from reactive arthritis
    - SI joint disease is usually bilateral (50%)
    - Predilection for upper extremities (especially DIP, PIP joints)
- Etiology-Pathogenesis
    - o Psoriatic arthritis arises in conjunction with psoriasis
    - o Reactive arthritis usually follows prior bacterial infection
- Epidemiology
    - o AS – 95% HLA – B27 positive; M >> F
        - Idiopathic, but known association with inflammatory bowel disease (IBD), iritis, aortitis, upper lobe pulmonary fibrosis
    - o Reactive arthritis – 80% HLA – B27 positive; M >> F
        - Occurs following non-gonococcal urethritis or bacillary dysentery
    - o Psoriatic arthritis – 50% HLA-B27 positive; M = F
        - Approximately 10 to 20% of psoriasis patients develop arthritis

Gross Pathologic-Surgical Features
- Spinal ankylosis predisposes patients to unusual two or three column unstable spine fractures
- Fractures heal with exuberant bone formation

Clinical Issues

Presentation
- AS – insidious onset of stiff back pain; SI joint involved first
    - o May develop cauda equina syndrome, with remodeling of lumbar canal (see Dural Ectasia Title)
- Reactive – classic triad of urethritis/cervicitis, conjunctivitis, arthritis
    - o Back and heel pain, balanitis common
- Psoriatic – predominant upper extremity arthritis in context of patient with psoriasis
    - o In 10% arthritis precedes skin changes
- Patients with IBD (ulcerative colitis, Crohn's disease), Whipple's disease, or bacillary dysentery infection (Salmonella, Shigella, Yersinia) may develop arthritis indistinguishable from reactive or psoriatic arthritis

Treatment
- Conservative anti-inflammatory management, immunomodulation

Prognosis
- Variable; usually progressive

Selected References
1. Luong AA et al: Imaging of the seronegative spondyloarthropathies. Curr Rheumatol Rep 2(4): 288-96, 2000
2. Braun JM et al: Radiologic diagnosis and pathology of the spondyloarthropathies. Rheum Dis Clin North Am 24(4): 697-735, 1998
3. Deesomchok U et al: Clinical comparison of patients with ankylosing spondylitis, Reiter's syndrome and psoriatic arthtitis. J Med Assoc Thai 76(2): 61-70, 1993

Foraminal Disc Extrusion

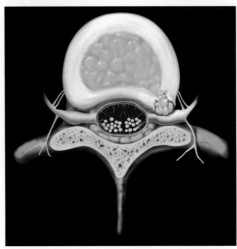

Axial illustration at the intervertebral disc level of the lumbar spine depicts a left foraminal disc extrusion, compressing the ipsilateral exiting nerve root. Anular tear is evident.

Key Facts
- Definition: Extruded disc material within the neural foramen
- Classic imaging appearance: Soft-tissue mass extending from the parent disc, effacing the perineural fat in the neural foramen
- Other key facts
  - Up to 10% of all disc herniations
  - Usually more symptomatic compared to other disc herniations
    - Irritation and/or impingement of the exiting nerve root in the narrow confines of the neural foramen
  - Most common at L3-4 and L4-5 levels
  - Typical "mushroom" appearance of central or subarticular disc extrusion not present
    - Restricted by the neural foramen
  - May not be detected by myelography
  - Location of disc herniation
    - 2001 ASNR, ASSR, and NASS consensus statement on lumbar disc terminology
    - Central, ipsilateral central, subarticular, foraminal, extra-foraminal (or far lateral) on axial imaging
    - Discal, infrapedicular, suprapedicular, or pedicular on sagittal imaging

Imaging Findings
General Features
- Best imaging clue
  - Obliterated perineural fat in the neural foramen on parasagittal images
  - Contiguity with the parent disc
CT Findings
- Disc density material within the neural foramen

Foraminal Disc Extrusion

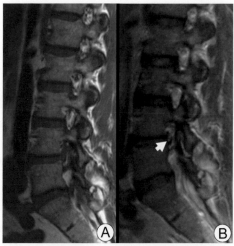

Sagittal T1WI (A) and T2WI (B) of the lumbar spine demonstrate foraminal disc extrusion at L4-5. The extruded material is isointense to the parent disc on T1, but hyperintense on T2. The exiting L4 nerve root is compressed. In addition, a foraminal anular tear is present (arrow).

- No enhancement, or
- Peripheral enhancement
- Other evidence of degenerative spondylosis

MR Findings
- T1WI: Isointense to parent disc
- T2WI: Iso-, hypo-, or hyperintense to parent disc
  - Depending on the hydration status of the extruded disc
- Absent or peripheral enhancement after intravenous gadolinium
- Variable extent of impingement of the exiting nerve root
  - May show postgadolinium enhancement

Imaging Recommendations
- Careful evaluation of parasagittal images for foraminal mass

Differential Diagnosis

Schwannoma
- Enlarged neural foramen due to chronic remodeling
- "Dumbbell" appearance on axial imaging
- Diffuse postcontrast enhancement
  - Unless necrosis present

Spinal Nerve Root Diverticulum
- Cerebral spinal fluid intensity on all sequences
- No enhancement
- Opacification on CT myelography

Large Facet Osteophyte
- Hypointense on T1WI and T2WI
- Contiguous with the facet joint
- Osseous density on CT

Pathology

<u>General</u>
- General Path Comments
  - Composed of a combination of nucleus pulposus, fragmented anulus, cartilage, and fragmented apophyseal bone
- Embryology-Anatomy
  - Nucleus pulposus centrally
    - Gelatinous material with high water content and few collagen fibers
    - Water content diminishes with age, replaced by fibrocartilage and fibrosis
  - Anulus fibrosus peripherally
    - Composed of fibrocartilage, with collagen fibers in concentric lamellae
    - Peripheral attachment to the longitudinal ligaments (anuloligamentous complex)
- Etiology-Pathogenesis
  - Degenerative or posttraumatic breach in the anulus
  - Disc material extends through the defect
- Epidemiology
  - Fifth decade of life or older

Clinical Issues

<u>Presentation</u>
- Radicular symptoms
  - Pain in a dermatomal distribution
  - Muscle weakness
  - L3 nerve root affected at L3-4 level
  - L4 nerve root affected at L4-5 level

<u>Natural History</u>
- May stabilize or resolve spontaneously

<u>Treatment</u>
- Bed rest and analgesic medications
  - No or minimal neurological impairment
- Discectomy if conservative treatment fails or neurological deficits present

<u>Prognosis</u>
- Favorable outcome

Selected References
1. Consensus statement on nomenclature and classification of lumbar disc pathology by NASS, ASSR, and ASNR. 2001
2. Lejeune JP: Foraminal lumbar disc herniation: Experience with 83 patients. Spine 19:1905-08, 1994
3. Osborn AG et al: CT/MR spectrum of far lateral and anterior lumbosacral disc herniations. AJNR 9:775-8, 1988

INFECTIONS

Tuberculous Spondylitis

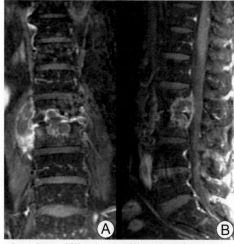

Gadolinium enhanced coronal (A) and sagittal (B) T1WI with fat saturation demonstrate an intraosseous abscess spanning the L2 and L3 vertebral bodies with epidural extension. The intervertebral disc is involved. A right psoas abscess is also present.

Key Facts
- Synonym: Pott's disease
- Definition: Tuberculous infection of the spine
- Classic imaging appearance
  - Vertebral gibbus deformity in late tuberculous spondylitis
  - Osteomyelitis involving multiple (non)contiguous vertebral bodies
  - Collapsed disc
  - Large paraspinal abscesses out of proportion to the degree of vertebral destruction or clinical symptoms
- Other key facts
  - Rising incidence of tuberculosis in the past two decades
  - Tuberculous spondylitis in less than 1% of patients with tuberculosis
  - Concomitant pulmonary tuberculosis in about 10% of patients
  - Compared to pyogenic spondylitis
    - Peak incidence in the third and fourth decades of life, compared to sixth and seventh decades
    - Predilection for the thoracolumbar junction versus the lower lumbar spine
    - Initial infection in the anterior vertebral body versus subchondral bone adjacent to the endplate
    - Gradual, insidious onset of symptoms
    - Posterior element involvement more common
    - Disc space may be preserved
    - Soft-tissue calcifications
    - Dissecting paravertebral abscesses over considerable distance

Imaging Findings
General Features
- Best imaging clue: Psoas abscess with calcifications

Tuberculous Spondylitis

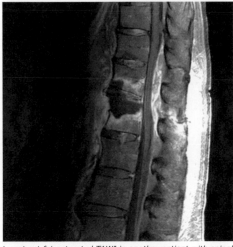

Sagittal post-contrast fat-saturated T1WI in another patient with spinal TB shows a non-enhancing area involving the T12 and L1 vertebral bodies and the intervening disc. The disc height is preserved. A posterior epidural enhancing phlegmon extends from T11 to L1, compressing the conus medullaris.

CT Findings
- Bony destruction, beginning in the anterior portion of the vertebral body
- Rib involvement in advanced cases
- Bony fragments (sequestra)
- Calcifications of paravertebral abscesses

MR Findings
- Vertebral osteomyelitis hypointense on T1WI and hyperintense on T2WI or STIR
- Isolated involvement of the vertebral body or the posterior element may occur
- Intervertebral disc normal or collapsed with T2 hyperintensity
- Intraosseous and paravertebral abscesses better seen with intravenous gadolinium

Plain Film Findings
- Findings may not be present until weeks after the onset of infection
- Diffuse vertebral sclerosis and destruction
- Disc space loss
- Fusion across the disc space in late stage
- Associated spinal deformity

Imaging Recommendations
- Sagittal STIR or FSE T2 with fat saturation most sensitive for bone marrow edema and epidural involvement

Differential Diagnosis

Fungal Spondylitis
- Focal rather than diffuse vertebral involvement with preserved vertebral structure
- No posterior element involvement
- Multiple sites involved

- Disc space collapse with disc gas more common
- Epidural extension common but not paraspinal involvement

Spinal Metastases
- Difficult to distinguish from isolated tuberculous or fungal vertebral osteomyelitis
- Typically lack epidural or paraspinal abscess
- Disc space preserved
- Tissue diagnosis may be required

Pathology
General
- Etiology-Pathogenesis
  o Initial inoculum in the anterior vertebral body with spread to (non)adjacent vertebral bodies beneath the longitudinal ligaments
  o Sparing of the intervertebral disc thought to be due to a lack of proteolytic enzymes
  o Hematogenous, paraspinal, or subarachnoid dissemination of disease also occurs
- Epidemiology
  o Third and fourth decades of life

Microscopic Features
- Caseating granulomas
- Acid fast bacilli

Clinical Issues
Presentation
- Chronic back pain
- Focal tenderness and kyphosis
- Fever
- Paraparesis
- Sensory disturbance
- Sphincter dysfunction

Natural History
- Vertebral collapse
- Irreversible neurologic deficits
- Death

Treatment
- Long term antibiotics for at least one year
- Surgical decompression, abscess drainage, and stabilization

Prognosis
- Favorable outcome with resolution of symptoms
- One-third of the patients with significant remaining deficits in one series

Selected References
1. Nussbaum ES et al: Spinal tuberculosis: a diagnostic and management challenge. J Neurosurg 83:243-7, 1995
2. Sharif HS et al: Granulomatous spinal infections: MR imaging. Radiology 177:101-7, 1990
3. Smith AS et al: MR imaging characteristics of tuberculous spondylitis vs vertebral osteomyelitis. AJNR 10:619-25, 1989

Pyogenic Spondylitis

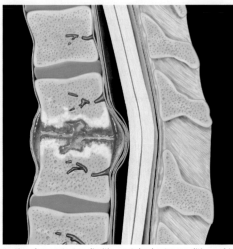

Sagittal illustration demonstrates discitis, vertebral osteomyelitis, and intervertebral abscess with epidural and pre-vertebral extension.

Key Facts
- Synonym: Discitis and vertebral osteomyelitis
- Definition: Infection of the vertebral bodies and the intervening disc
- Classic imaging appearance
  - Narrowed disc space with T2 hyperintensity
  - Bone marrow changes, hypointense on T1WI and hyperintense on T2WI, in the adjacent vertebral bodies
  - Endplate erosions
- Other key facts
  - Predilection for lower lumbar spine
  - MRI is the imaging modality of choice
  - Plain film negative up to 2 to 8 weeks after the onset of symptoms

Imaging Findings
General Features
- Best imaging clue
  - Vertebral marrow T1 hypointensity with loss of endplate definition on both sides of the disc
  - Disc T2 hyperintensity
  - Associated soft tissue inflammation
CT Findings
- Axial imaging good for endplate osteolytic/osteosclerotic changes and epidural and paraspinal abscesses
- Sagittal reformation good for disc space narrowing in addition to endplate destructive changes
MR Findings
- Signal abnormality abutting the disc in adjacent vertebral bodies
  - Hypointense on T1WI
  - Vivid enhancement with gadolinium
  - Hyperintense or isointense on T2WI
  - Hyperintense on fat saturated T2 or STIR imaging

Pyogenic Spondylitis

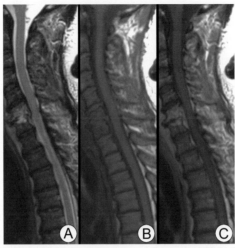

Sagittal T2WI (A) and T1WI (B) reveal narrowed disc space at C6-7 with end-plate erosion. Marrow changes are hyperintense on T2WI and hypointense on T1WI, with post-gadolinium enhancement (C). Pre-vertebral and epidural enhancing soft tissue is also present, narrowing the canal (C).

- Disc space narrowing
  - Hypointense on T1WI
  - Variable, typically hyperintense on T2WI
- Endplate cortical bone erosion
- Enhancing disc after intravenous gadolinium
- Associated paraspinal and epidural phlegmon or abscess
  - Better seen with gadolinium

Plain Film Findings
- Negative up to 2 to 8 weeks after the onset of symptoms
- Disc space narrowing
- Endplate erosions and collapse
- Bony sclerosis and fusion across the disc space late in disease course

Imaging Recommendations
- Sagittal STIR or FSE T2 with fat saturation most sensitive for bone marrow edema and epidural involvement

Differential Diagnosis

Degenerative Spondylosis
- Most common mimic
- Normal erythrocyte sedimentation rate and/or C reactive protein very helpful
- Disc desiccation usually present
  - Hypointense on T1WI and (usually) on T2WI as well
- Vertebral endplates often preserved
- Presence of Schmorl's nodes
- Disc space aspiration in difficult cases, e.g. when hyperintense on T2WI

Spinal Metastases
- Difficult to distinguish from isolated tuberculous or fungal vertebral osteomyelitis

Pyogenic Spondylitis

- Typically lack epidural or paraspinal abscess
- Disc space preserved
- Tissue diagnosis maybe required

Spondyloarthropathy Related to Chronic Hemodialysis
- Extensive, multifocal destructive changes
- Other signs of renal osteodystrophy
- Lack of soft tissue component
- Clinical history
- Presence of amyloid on biopsy

Pathology
General
- Etiology-Pathogenesis
  - o Staphylococcus aureus is the most common pathogen
  - o Bacteremia from an extraspinal primary source
    - ▪ Most common route of infection
    - ▪ Vascularized subchondral bone adjacent to the endplate seeded primarily
    - ▪ Secondary infection of the intervertebral disc and the adjacent vertebral body
  - o Other routes of infection
    - ▪ Direct inoculation from penetrating trauma, surgical intervention, or diagnostic procedures
    - ▪ Extension from adjacent infection in the paraspinal soft tissues
- Epidemiology
  - o Peak incidence in the six and seventh decades

Clinical Issues
Presentation
- Acute or chronic back pain
- Focal tenderness
- Fever, elevated erythrocyte sedimentation rate, C reactive protein, and white cell count
- Paraparesis
- Sensory disturbance

Natural History
- Vertebral collapse
- Irreversible neurological deficits
- Death

Treatment
- Long term antibiotics for a total of six to eight weeks
- Surgical decompression in neurologically compromised patients with epidural abscess

Prognosis
- Favorable outcome with resolution of symptoms with prompt diagnosis and treatment

Selected References
1. Dagirmanjian A et al: MR Imaging of Vertebral Osteomyelitis Revisited. AJR 167:1539-43, 1996
2. Thrush A et al: MR Imaging of Infectious Spondylitis. AJNR 11:1171-80, 1990
3. Smith AS et al: MR Imaging Characteristics of Tuberculous Spondylitis vs Vertebral Osteomyelitis. AJR 153:399-405, 1989

Septic Facet Joint Arthritis

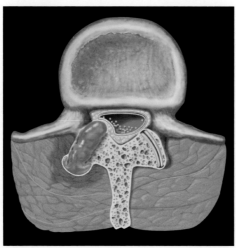

Axial illustration of the lumbar spine depicts an abscess eroding and widening the right facet joint. There is epidural extension, distorting the thecal sac. Posterior paraspinal extension is also present, surrounded by inflammation.

Key Facts
- Synonym: Septic facet arthritis
- Definition: Hematogenous infection of the facet joint
- Classic imaging appearance: Enhancing facet joint with paraspinal or epidural phlegmon or abscess
- Other key facts
  - Rare, 4% of infectious spondylitis in one series
  - Most common (97%) in the lumbar spine
  - Complicated by epidural abscess in 25% of the cases
  - Erythrocyte sedimentation rate and C-reactive protein always elevated
  - Difficult to distinguish from spondylodiscitis clinically
  - Plain films may be negative up to 2 to 8 weeks after the onset of infection

Imaging Findings
General Features
- Best imaging clue: Unilateral facet joint T2 hyperintensity with abnormal marrow signal abutting the joint

CT Findings
- Slightly expanded facet joint with fluid density
- Mixed lytic/sclerotic osseous changes
- Contiguous epidural or posterior paraspinal phlegmonous inflammation or abscess

MR Findings
- T2 hyerintensity within the facet joint
  - Hypointense on T1WI
    - Enhances after intravenous gadolinium
- Marrow signal alteration abutting the facet joint
  - Hypointense on T1WI
  - Hyperintense on fat saturated T2WI or STIR

Septic Facet Joint Arthritis

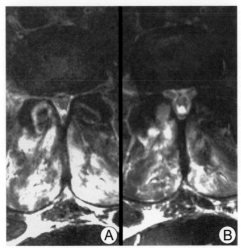

Axial T2WI (A) of the lumbar spine demonstrates asymmetric T2 hyperintensity in the right facet joint. More caudally (B), the joint appears expanded with hyperintensity in the adjacent posterior paraspinal soft tissue.

- o Postgadolinium enhancement
- o Cortical erosive changes
- Enhancing soft tissue or peripherally enhancing fluid collection
  - o Contiguous with the facet joint
  - o Epidural or posterior paraspinal extension

Technetium 99m Bone Scintigraphy or Gallium Citrate Imaging
- Nonspecific uptake
  - o Degenerative, infectious, posttraumatic, versus neoplastic
- More laterally located and vertically oriented uptake compared to spondylodiscitis

Imaging Recommendations
- Sagittal STIR or FSE T2 with fat saturation most sensitive for bone marrow edema and epidural involvement
- Postgadolinium T1WI with fat saturation better delineates the extent of epidural and paraspinal involvement

Differential Diagnosis
Facet Joint Arthropathy
- Facet hypertrophy
  - o Usually with associated ligamentum flavum hypertrophy
- Symmetric bilaterally
  - o Unless scoliosis present
- No marrow signal changes or associated soft tissue or fluid collection
- Normal erythrocyte sedimentation rate and C-reactive protein

Facet Synovial Cyst
- Cyst wall thin and well defined
- No marrow signal abnormality
- Associated facet and ligamentum flavum hypertrophy
- Normal erythrocyte sedimentation rate and C-reactive protein

Septic Facet Joint Arthritis

Pathology

General
- Etiology-Pathogenesis
  - Staphylococcus aureus is the most common pathogen
  - Predisposing factors
    - Intravenous drug abuse
    - Diabetes mellitus and other chronic medical illnesses
  - Bacteremia from an extraspinal primary source
    - Most common route of infection
    - GU or GI tract, lungs, or cutaneous source
  - Other routes of infection
    - Direct inoculation from penetrating trauma, surgical intervention, or diagnostic procedures
    - Extension from adjacent infection in the paraspinal soft tissues
- Epidemiology
  - Sixth decade of life or older
  - Younger population with intravenous drugs involved

Clinical Issues

Presentation
- Acute or chronic back pain
- Focal tenderness
- Fever, elevated erythrocyte sedimentation rate, C reactive protein, and white count
- Neurological impairment with extra-facet extension and epidural involvement
  - Radiculopathy
  - Paraparesis
  - Sensory disturbance
  - Sphincter dysfunction

Natural History
- Osseous destruction and progressive neurological deterioration
- Sepsis and death

Treatment
- Intravenous antibiotics
- Percutaneous joint drainage
- Decompressive laminectomy when epidural abscess and neurological deficits present

Prognosis
- Favorable outcome with intravenous antibiotics alone
- Success rate slightly improved if combined with percutaneous drainage

Selected References
1. Muffoletto AJ et al: Hematogenous pyogenic facet joint infection. Spine 26:1570-6, 2001
2. Rombauts PA et al: Septic arthritis of a lumbar facet joint caused by Staphylococcus aureus. Spine 25:1736-8, 2000
3. Ergan M et al: Septic arthritis of lumbar facet joint. A review of six cases. Rev Rhum Engl Ed 64:386-95, 1997

Epidural Abscess

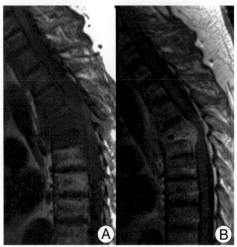

Sagittal T1WI pre- (A) and post-gadolinium (B) images through the thoracic spine demonstrate T4-5 discitis and vertebral osteomyelitis with associated diffusely enhancing epidural phlegmon, narrowing the central canal.

Key Facts
- Definition: Extradural spinal infection with abscess formation
- Classic imaging appearance
  - Peripheral enhancing epidural collection
- Other key facts
  - Early diagnosis and prompt treatment improve prognosis
  - Contrast enhanced MRI is the imaging modality of choice
  - Common association with vertebral osteomyelitis

Imaging Findings
General Features
- Best imaging clue: Findings of discitis and vertebral osteomyelitis, with adjacent enhancing epidural phlegmon or peripherally enhancing fluid collection

MR Findings
- Focal or diffuse epidural soft-tissue intensity
  - Isointense to hypointense on T1WI
  - Hyperintense on T2WI
  - Homogeneously or heterogeneously enhancing phlegmon
  - Peripherally enhancing liquid abscess
- Anterior spinal location when arising from adjacent discitis and vertebral osteomyelitis
- Posterior spinal location when caused by bacteremia, or septic facet arthritis
- Enhancing prominent anterior epidural veins or the basivertebral venous plexus above or below the abscess
- Diffuse dural enhancement with more extensive disease
- Various degree of encroachment on the central canal
- Signal alteration in the spinal cord from
  - Cord compression

Epidural Abscess

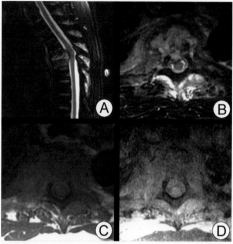

Sagittal T2WI with fat saturation (A) and axial T2WI (B) demonstrate the hyperintense epidural phlegmon. In addition, axial T1 pre- (C) and post-gadolinium (D) images reveal paraspinal enhancing inflammatory soft tissue.

- o Cord ischemia
- o Direct infection
- Persistent epidural enhancement without mass effect on follow-up MR imaging
  - o Probable sterile granulation tissue or fibrosis
  - o Correlation with erythrocyte sedimentation rate for disease activity

Differential Diagnosis
Epidural Metastasis
- Contiguous lesion involving the adjacent vertebral body
- Expansion of the involved vertebral body
- Sparing of the spinal column in some cases
- Diffuse enhancement

Epidural Hematoma
- Isointense to hypointense on T2WI
- No post-gadolinium enhancement

Extruded Disc
- Associated parent disc protrusion, degeneration
- More focal appearance, attached to the parent disc
- Often isointense on T2WI

Pathology
General
- Etiology-Pathogenesis
  - o Staphylococcus aureus is the most common pathogen (57-73%)
  - o Mycobacterium tuberculosis is the next most frequent cause
  - o Fungal infection rare, but more common in the immunocompromised host
  - o Predisposing factors
    - Intravenous drug abuse

- Immunocompromised state
- Diabetes mellitus and other chronic medical illnesses
- o Often arises from adjacent discitis and vertebral osteomyelitis
- o Other routes of infection
  - Hematogenous from the GU or GI tract, lungs, or cutaneous source
  - Direct from penetrating trauma, surgical intervention, or diagnostic procedures
  - Extension from adjacent infection in the paraspinal soft tissues
- o Extension of epidural involvement by tracking beneath the posterior longitudinal ligament
- o Tuberculous infection spreads under the anterior ligament, often sparing the disc
- Epidemiology
  - o 0.2 to 2 cases per 10,000
  - o Peak incidence in the sixth and seventh decades

Microscopic Features
- Leukocytes, micro-organisms, cellular debris, and granulation tissue

Clinical Issues
Presentation
- Acute or subacute spinal pain and tenderness
- Fever
- Weakness and paresthesia
- Loss of bladder and bowel control

Natural History
- Irreversible neurologic deficit and death if untreated or delay in treatment

Treatment
- Emergent surgical decompression with drainage of abscess when neurologically compromised
- Early empiric antibiotics with broad spectrum coverage until causative pathogen isolated
- Organism specific intravenous antibiotics followed by long term parenteral antibiotics

Prognosis
- Determined by
  - o Initial neurologic deficits
  - o Co-morbidities
  - o Early diagnosis and institution of treatment
    - Shorter duration between the onset of neurological deficits and the time of surgical intervention predictive of a better neurologic outcome

Selected References
1. Mackenzie AR et al: Spinal epidural abscess: the importance of early diagnosis and treatment. J Neurol Neurosurg Psychiatry 65:209-12, 1998
2. Numaguchi Y et al: Spinal Epidural Abscess: Evaluation with Gadolinium-enhanced MR Imaging. RadioGraphics 13:545-59, 1993
3. Nussbaum ES et al: Spinal Epidural Abscess: A Report of 40 Cases and Review. Surg Neurol 38:225-31, 1992

Paraspinal Abscess

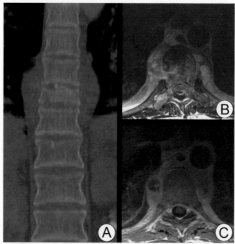

Coronal CT reformation of the thoracic spine (A) demonstrates bilateral paraspinal masses, which are predominantly hyperintense on axial T2WI (B). The vertebral body, partially collapsed on CT, has abnormal signal intensity. Axial T1WI with gadolinium (C) reveals foci of nonenhancement, consistent with abscesses.

Key Facts
- Definition: Infection of the soft tissues surrounding the spine
- Classic imaging appearance: Peripherally-enhancing paraspinal collection
- Most often associated with adjacent spondylodiscitis

Imaging Findings
General Features
- Best imaging clue: Findings of discitis and vertebral osteomyelitis, with adjacent enhancing phlegmon or peripherally-enhancing collection
CT Findings
- Paravertebral soft-tissue cavitary mass with surrounding fascial blurring
- Psoas or posterior vertebral muscle involvement
  - Diffuse enhancement
  - Low-density collection
    - Thick and irregular peripheral enhancement
  - Calcified psoas abscesses characteristic of tuberculous infection
- Direct extension from vertebral osteomyelitis or
- Secondary involvement of the spine
- May see appendicitis or Crohn's disease in the abdomen as the primary source of infection
MR Findings
- Enlarged psoas or posterior vertebral muscles
  - Focal or diffuse
  - Hypo- to isointense on T1WI
  - Hyperintense on T2WI
  - Postgadolinium diffuse or ringlike enhancement
- Anterior paravertebral soft-tissue mass
  - Variable cranial-caudal dimension
  - Amorphous, infiltrative

Paraspinal Abscess

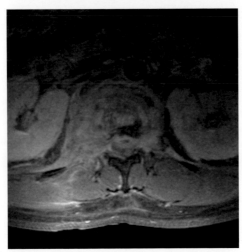

Axial postgadolinium T1WI with fat saturation at the level of the renal hilum in another patient shows right, greater than left, enhancing paraspinal and epidural phlegmon, associated with discitis and vertebral osteomyelitis.

- o Intermediate signal intensity on T1WI
- o Hyperintense on T2WI
- o Diffuse enhancement
- o Foci of nonenhancement suggestive of liquefaction
- Features of spondylitis
  - o Possible epidural extension

Imaging Recommendations
- T2WI with fat suppression or STIR improves detection of early paraspinal inflammation

Differential Diagnosis
Neoplasm, Primary or Metastatic
- Soft-tissue mass more discrete
- Diffuse post-gadolinium enhancement
  - o Large mass may contain necrotic elements
- Lymphoma may have intermediate signal intensity on T2WI
- Variable involvement of the spine

Retroperitoneal Hematoma
- Typically more diffuse
- No enhancement
- May see fluid-fluid level if anti-coagulated

Pathology
General
- Etiology-Pathogenesis
  - o Staphylococcus aureus and Mycobacterium tuberculosis are the most common pathogens
  - o Fungal infection rare, but more common in the immunocompromised host

- o Predisposing factors
  - ▪ Intravenous drug abuse
  - ▪ Immunocompromised state
  - ▪ Diabetes mellitus and other chronic medical illnesses
- o Direct extension from adjacent infection
  - ▪ Spondylodiscitis
  - ▪ Appendicitis
  - ▪ Inflammatory bowel disease
  - ▪ Perinephric abscess
- o Transcutaneous infection of the deep tissue
  - ▪ Trauma
  - ▪ Needles or catheters
  - ▪ Surgery
- o Hematogenous spread from distant sites

<u>Microscopic Features</u>
- Leukocytes, micro-organisms, cellular debris, and granulation tissue

Clinical Issues
<u>Presentation</u>
- Fever
- Back pain and tenderness
- Lower extremity pain
- If epidural component present
  - o Weakness
  - o Paresthesia
  - o Sphincter dysfunction

<u>Natural History</u>
- Depends on host immune response
  - o May be contained with early treatment
- Overwhelming sepsis
  - o Leading to death in debilitated host
- Progressive neurological impairment if spondylitis present

<u>Treatment</u>
- Intravenous antibiotics
- Analgesic medications
- Percutaneous catheter drainage
- Surgical debridement

<u>Prognosis</u>
- Dependent on
  - o Co-morbidities
  - o Extent of spinal involvement
  - o Degree of neurological compromise

Selected References
1. Hill JS et al: A Staphylococcus aureus paraspinal abscess associated with epidural analgesia in labour. Anaesthesia 56:871-8, 2001
2. Dagirmanjian A et al: MR imaging of vertebral osteomyelitis revisited. AJR 167:1539-43, 1996
3. Nussbaum ES et al: Spinal tuberculosis: a diagnostic and management challenge. J Neurosurg 83:243-7, 1995

Human Immunodeficiency Virus-HIV

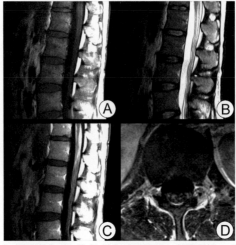

CMV polyradiculitis (AIDS patient). (A, B) Sagittal T1WI and T2WI show mild thickening of the proximal cauda equina. (C) Sagittal T1WI with contrast shows avid pial and cauda equina enhancement. (D) Axial T1WI after contrast confirms abnormal nerve root enhancement.

Key Facts
- Synonym(s): HIV myelitis, HIV myelopathy
- Definition: Primary HIV myelitis may be solitary or accompanied by opportunistic infection or neoplasm
- Classic imaging appearance: HIV myelitis is characterized by spinal cord enlargement and T2 hyperintensity; may show patchy enhancement
- HIV myelitis is rare
- AIDS patients at increased risk for opportunistic infections/neoplasm
  - CMV, tuberculosis (TB), fungi, parasites (Toxoplasma), and lymphoma
  - More commonly seen than primary HIV myelitis

Imaging Findings
General Features
- Best imaging clue: T2 hyperintense spinal cord lesion in AIDS patient
- Imaging studies for HIV myelitis may be normal
  - Abnormal studies show non-specific T2 hyperintensity
- Opportunistic infections, lymphoma usually more specific in appearance
CT Findings
- HIV – normal or cord enlargement
- CMV – usually negative; may see subtle nerve root enhancement
- TB – destructive spondylitis with severe gibbus deformity
  - Begins in anterior vertebral body, **relatively** spares the disc space
  - May see bilateral calcified paraspinal masses
- Lymphoma – destructive lesion; enhancing paraspinal or intradural component
MR Findings
- HIV – normal or cord enlargement with T2 hyperintensity (indistinguishable from transverse myelitis of other causes)
- CMV – normal or mild root thickening on unenhanced T1WI and T2WI
  - Cauda equina/conus pial enhancement

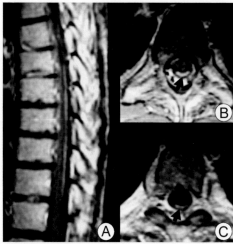

Lymphoma (AIDS patient). Sagittal T1WI (A) post contrast shows intradural enhancing tumor along dorsal cord. Axial T1WI (B, C) post contrast confirms intradural location (arrows) along dorsal cord surface.

- TB – protean MRI appearance
  - Destructive spondylitis, severe gibbus deformity, paraspinal masses
  - Dura-arachnoid complex enhancement
  - Nodular enhancing intramedullary tuberculoma
  - Cord expansion, diffuse T2 hyperintensity due to vasculitis, myelitis
- Toxoplasma – focally enhancing cord mass mimicking an intramedullary tumor
- Lymphoma – destructive lesion with enhancing paraspinal and/or intradural component

Imaging Recommendations
- Sagittal, axial T1WI and T2WI
- Sagittal and axial post contrast T1WI
- CT can confirm presence of paraspinal calcification with TB

Differential Diagnosis
Transverse Myelitis
- Cord enlargement, paralysis
- Nonspecific end result of cord infection, post vaccination or multiple sclerosis demyelination, infarction, radiation myelitis, paraneoplastic syndrome, or collagen–vascular disease

Pathology
General
- General Path Comments
  - Vacuolar myelopathy, probably related to direct HIV injury of neurons
  - Posterior and lateral column demyelination
  - 15% to 30% of adult AIDS patients demonstrate CMV intranuclear inclusions in spinal cord, nerves, and retina
- Etiology-Pathogenesis
  - HIV myelopathy – direct HIV infection

o Opportunistic infections, lymphoma occur later with T cell depletion
- Epidemiology
  o HIV myelopathy – imaging manifestations rare
  o TB –AIDS epidemic is responsible for recrudescence of U.S. tuberculosis cases (especially spinal TB)
    ▪ Hematogenous spread from pulmonary source
    ▪ 75% of cases in patients under 30 years of age

Gross Pathologic-Surgical Features
- TB
  o Massive bone destruction, kyphosis, relative disc sparing
  o Congested meninges with inflammatory exudates
  o Tuberculoma may be anywhere within dural sac
- Lymphoma
  o Destructive bone mass; frequently with paraspinal and/or epidural enhancing mass; less frequently can be intradural

Microscopic Features
- HIV – vacuolar myelopathy, posterior and lateral column demyelination
- CMV – characteristic intranuclear inclusions
- TB – thick, gelatinous, inflammatory exudate coats nerves, leptomeninges

Clinical Issues

Presentation
- Primary HIV neurologic manifestations include encephalopathy, myelopathy, peripheral neuropathy, and myopathy
- CMV polyradiculopathy – subacute progressive weakness, hyporeflexia, mild ascending sensory symptoms
  o Relentlessly progresses unless treated
- TB – cord compression with neurologic deficit

Treatment
- HIV – highly active retroviral therapy (HART)
- CMV – anti-viral therapy (Gancyclovir)
- TB – anti-tuberculosis antibiotics; surgery for cord compression or correction of gibbus deformity
- Lymphoma – surgical decompression/radiation; chemotherapy

Prognosis
- Variable depending on etiological agent
  o TB may improve with therapy and/or surgery
  o HIV, CMV may stabilize but not improve following therapy
  o Lymphoma has poor prognosis

Selected References
1. Di Rocco A: Diseases of the spinal cord in human immunodeficiency virus infection. Semin Neurol 19(2):151-5, 1999
2. Thurnher MM et al: Diagnostic imaging of infections and neoplasms affecting the spine in patients with AIDS. Neuroimaging Clin N Am 7(2):341-57, 1997
3. Quencer RM et al: Spinal cord lesions in patients with AIDS. Neuroimaging Clin N Am 7(2): 359-73, 1997

Spinal Meningitis

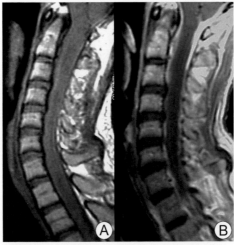

Sagittal T1WI (A) of the cervical spine demonstrates indistinctness of the subarachnoid space. After intravenous gadolinium (B), there is diffuse leptomeningeal enhancement, extending into the posterior fossa.

Key Facts
- Definition: Infection of the spinal cord leptomeninges and the subarachnoid space
- Classic imaging appearance: Smooth or nodular leptomeningeal enhancement on contrast enhanced MRI
- Other key facts
  - Pyogenic, fungal, or viral infection
  - CT or MRI most often negative at the time of diagnosis
  - Secondarily from intracranial meningitis or infectious spondylitis
  - Medical emergency requiring prompt diagnosis and treatment

Imaging Findings
General Features
- Best imaging clue (if present): Meningeal enhancement, seen more often with tuberculous or fungal infections

CT Myelography Findings
- Block of cerebral spinal fluid
- Irregular contour of the thecal sac
- Nodular or band-like filling defects adherent to the cord surface
- Thickened nerve roots
- Focal or diffuse cord swelling

MR Findings
- Obliterated subarachnoid space on T1WI and T2WI
- Focal or diffuse cord swelling
  - Iso- to hypointense on T1WI
  - Hyperintense on T2WI
- Diffuse or focal, smooth or nodular enhancement of the dura-arachnoid complex after intravenous gadolinium
- Enhancing nodules in the cauda equina

Spinal Meningitis

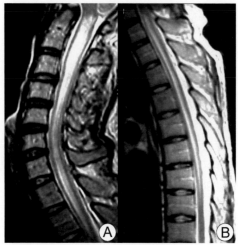

Sagittal T2WI of the cervical (A) and thoracic spine (B) in the same patient reveals diffuse intramedullary hyperintensity, consistent with cord ischemia.

- May see leptomeningeal enhancement in the posterior fossa when imaging the cervical spine
- May be complicated by subdural empyema
- Segmental or nodular intramedullary enhancement may be present

Imaging Recommendations
- Intravenous gadolinium increases the sensitivity in detecting meningeal disease

Differential Diagnosis
Carcinomatous or Lymphomatous Meningitis
- History of intra- or extracranial primary neoplasm
- No signs of infection

Sarcoidosis
- Concurrent systemic manifestations
- Focal intramedullary areas of enhancement more common

Pathology
General
- Etiology-Pathogenesis
  - Extension of intracranial meningitis or infectious spondylitis
  - History of trauma or surgical procedures
  - Acute inflammatory exudate in the subarachnoid space after the offending organisms enter the cerebral spinal fluid
  - Spinal cord swelling and focal enhancement likely to due ischemia from vasculitis, venous congestion, and/or infectious myelitis
- Epidemiology
  - Common bacteria include Streptococcus pneumoniae, Neisseria meningitides, and Hemophilus influenzae
  - Atypical infections include tuberculosis, coccidioidomycosis, cryptococcosis, and aspergillosis

Spinal Meningitis

<u>Microscopic Features</u>
- Cellular debris, inflammatory cells, and micro-organisms
- Tuberculous meningitis: Small tubercles consist of epithelioid cells, Langerhans' giant cells, and foci of caseation

Clinical Issues
<u>Presentation</u>
- Acute onset of fever, headache, and altered level of consciousness
- Symptoms less acute in tuberculous or fungal meningitis
- Generalized convulsions
- Neck stiffness
- Paraparesis
- Paresthesia
- Gait disturbance
- Urinary bladder dysfunction

<u>Natural History</u>
- Progressive neurologic deterioration, potentially permanent, leading to death

<u>Treatment</u>
- Broad spectrum intravenous antibiotics while waiting for culture results
- Organism specific intravenous antibiotics
- Oral rifampin for close contacts of the patient

<u>Prognosis</u>
- Excellent recovery without residual deficits if proper treatment begun early

Selected References
1. Post MD et al: Magnetic resonance imaging of spinal infection. Rheum Dis Clin North Am 17:773-94, 1991
2. Chang KH et al: Tuberculous arachnoiditis of the spine: Findings on Myelography, CT, and MR imaging. AJNR 10:1255-62, 1989

INFLAMMATORY AUTOIMMUNE

Guillain-Barre Syndrome

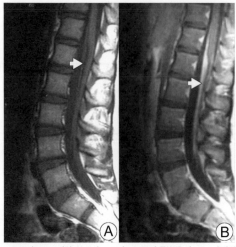

Guillain-Barre syndrome: (A) Unenhanced sagittal T1WI shows slightly thickened nerve roots (arrow). (B) Sagittal enhanced T1WI confirms avid enhancement of the thickened ventral nerve roots and surface of conus (arrow). (Case courtesy of Gregory L. Katzman, M.D.)

Key Facts
- Synonyms: Acute inflammatory demyelinating polyradiculoneuropathy
- Definition: Acute inflammatory demyelination of peripheral nerves, nerve roots, cranial nerves
- Classic imaging appearance: Diffuse enhancement of conus and cauda equina (with or without nerve root thickening)
- Most common cause of acute paralysis in Western countries
- Classically presents with "ascending paralysis"
  - Sensory loss common but less severe

Imaging Findings
General Features
- Best imaging clue: Smooth pial enhancement of the cauda equina and conus medullaris

CT Findings
- Normal except cauda equina and conus pia may enhance
- Difficult to diagnosis with CT

MR Findings
- Avid enhancement of the cauda equina/nerve roots and conus pia
- Nerve roots may be thickened

Imaging Recommendations
- Sagittal and axial T1WI without and with gadolinium contrast

Differential Diagnosis
Vasculitic Neuropathy
- Polyarteritis nodosa or Churg-Strauss most commonly
- Cranial nerves and respiratory nerves frequently spared

Acute Transverse Myelitis
- Cranial nerves always spared

Guillain-Barre Syndrome

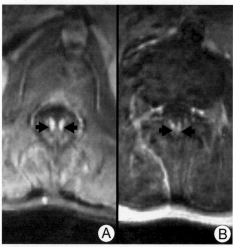

Guillain-Barre Syndrome. (A, B) Enhanced axial T1WIs confirm thickened, avidly enhancing nerve roots (arrows).

<u>Carcinomatous or Lymphomatous Meningitis</u>
- Enhancement is frequently more nodular than GBS
- Conus deposits frequently cause T2 signal abnormality

<u>Physiological Nerve Root Enhancement</u>
- Much more subtle enhancement of normal roots
- Absent clinical syndrome

Pathology
<u>General</u>
- General Path Comments
  - Lesions are scattered throughout peripheral nerves, nerve roots, cranial nerves
- Etiology-Pathogenesis
  - Inflammatory (postulated autoimmune or viral) demyelination; usually follows recent viral illness, C. jejuni infection, or vaccination
  - More tenuous association with preceding recent surgery or systemic illness
- Epidemiology
  - Incidence - 0.6 to 1.9 per 100,000 population
  - Affects all ages, races, socioeconomic status

<u>Microscopic Features</u>
- Focal segmental demyelination
- Perivascular and endoneural lymphocytic/monocytic infiltrates
- Axonal degeneration in conjunction with segmental demyelination in severe cases

Clinical Issues
<u>Presentation</u>
- Distal parasthesias rapidly followed by "ascending paralysis"
  - Frequently bilateral and symmetric
  - May require prolonged respiratory support in severe cases

Guillain-Barre Syndrome

- Autonomic disturbances
- Cranial nerve involvement common
  - Facial nerve involved in up to 50% of cases
  - Ophthalmoparesis in 10% to 20% of cases

Treatment
- Medical management with plasma exchange or intravenous gamma globulin
- No proven benefit from corticosteroid administration
- Intensive care management in severe cases

Prognosis
- Clinical nadir at 4 weeks
- Most patients somewhat better by 2 to 3 months
  - 50% have persistent symptoms at 1 year
  - Permanent deficits in 5% to 10%
- 2% to 10% relapse
  - 6% develop chronic course resembling CIDP (chronic inflammatory demyelinating polyneuropathy)

Selected References
1.   Cros D: Peripheral neuropathy. First ed. Philadelphia: Lippincott Williams & Wilkins, 2001
2.   Crino PB et al: Magnetic resonance imaging of the cauda equina in Guillain-Barre syndrome. Neurology 44(7): 1334-6, 1994
3.   Rowland L: Meritt's textbook of neurology. Eighth ed. Lea & Febiger: Philadelphia, 1989

Lumbar Arachnoiditis

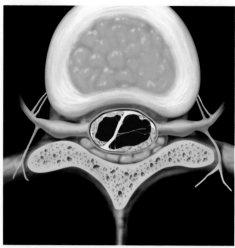

Axial illustration of the lumbar spine depicts nerve roots plastered to the periphery of the dural sac, demonstrating the "empty thecal sac" sign. Intrathecal adhesions are evident.

Key Facts
- Synonym: Chronic adhesive arachnoiditis
- Definition: Post-inflammatory adhesion and clumping of nerve roots, associated loculation of the subarachnoid space
- Classic imaging appearance
  - Absence of discrete nerve roots in the thecal sac
  - Large clump of nerve roots centrally within the thecal sac
  - "Empty thecal sac" sign
    - Peripheral thickening of the thecal sac
    - Central cerebral spinal fluid without nerve roots
  - Soft-tissue mass occupying most of the thecal sac
  - Blunted nerve root sleeves at myelography
- Other key facts
  - Uncommon entity
  - Cause of persistent pain in approximately 10% of post-laminectomy patients

Imaging Findings
General Features
- Best imaging clue: Absence of discrete nerve roots in the thecal sac
CT Myelogram Findings
- In addition to the classic imaging appearance
  - Intraspinal cysts and loculations
  - Rarely, calcifications of the nerve roots or the whole mass
MR Findings
- Spectrum ranging from clumping of two to three nerve roots to the classic imaging appearance
- Findings extend over at least two lumber vertebral bodies
- Presence of pantopaque from prior myelography

Lumbar Arachnoiditis

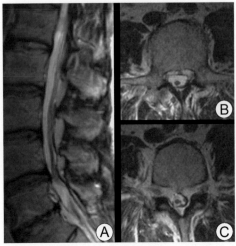

Lumbar arachnoiditis: Sagittal T2WI (A) demonstrates a conglomerate of lumbar nerve roots centrally within the thecal sac. Axial T2WI (B) confirms the centrally located cord-like nerve roots. In addition, peripherally clumped nerve roots are present (C).

- Evidence of prior lumbar surgery
- Variable degree of nerve root enhancement

Myelography Findings
- Obliterated nerve root sleeves
- Loss of nerve root shadow

Differential Diagnosis

Spinal Stenosis
- Clumped nerve roots
- Degenerative changes prominent

Intrathecal Neoplasm, Carcinomatous Meningitis, Leptomeningeal Spread
- More vigorous enhancement of nerve roots with focal nodules

Pathology

General
- Etiology-Pathogenesis
  - In the past, more commonly related to trauma or spinal meningitis
    - Tuberculous meningitis
    - Syphilis
  - Now more commonly associated with prior lumbar surgery
    - Especially when multiple or complicated
    - In combination with antecedent multiple or complicated spinal myelography, water or oil-based agents
  - Myelography alone elicits an intrathecal inflammatory response
    - Rarely leads to arachnoiditis
  - Intrathecal hemorrhage shown to irritate meninges in animal models
  - Common pathway of
    - Inflammatory cellular reaction
    - Fibrin deposition

Lumbar Arachnoiditis

- Perineural and leptomeningeal fibrosis
- Nerve roots adhering to one another and to the thecal sac
  - o Other causes
    - Subarachnoid hemorrhage
    - Spinal anesthesia
- Epidemiology
  - o < 1,000 cases reported in the literature over 50 years
  - o Clinical syndrome probably more common

Gross Pathologic-Surgical Features
- Inflammatory, collagenous mass
- Maybe calcified
- Posterior nerve roots involved more commonly

Microscopic Features
- Collagen formation
- Chronic lymphocytic infiltration
- Small areas of calcifications

Clinical Issues

Presentation
- No defining clinical symptomatology
- Simulates spinal stenosis and polyneuropathy
- Low back pain
- Radicular or non-radicular leg pain
- Paraparesis
- Bladder and bowel dysfunction

Natural History
- Symptoms usually static, but may fluctuate in severity
- Small percentage (1.8% in one series) with progressive neurological deficits

Treatment
- Intrathecal steroid injection
- Spinal cord stimulation
  - o Treatment of choice when pain is the predominant symptom
- Pain rehabilitation
- Laminectomy with microlysis of adhesions
  - o Reserved for patients with progressive neurological deficits

Prognosis
- Spinal cord stimulation
  - o Immediate success rate (pain relief) of > 70%
  - o Intermediate success rate of > 50%
  - o Long-term success rate of > 30%
- Microlysis of adhesions
  - o 50% initial success rate
  - o Decreases over time

Selected References
1. Long DM: Chronic adhesive spinal arachnoiditis: pathogenesis, prognosis, and treatment. Neurosurgery Quarterly 2:296-318, 1992
2. Delamarter RB et al: Diagnosis of lumbar arachnoiditis by magnetic resonance imaging. Spine 15:304-10, 1990
3. Ross JS et al: MR imaging of lumbar arachnoiditis. AJR 149:1025-32, 1987

Arachnoiditis Ossificans

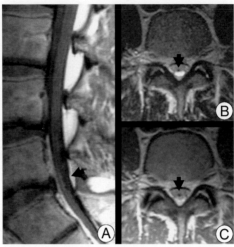

Sagittal T1WI of the lumbar spine (A) demonstrates a conglomerate of nerve roots in the thecal sac, consistent with arachnoiditis. A subtle linear hypointensity is present (arrow) at the level of L5-S1, which is confirmed on axial T2WI (arrow in B) and PDWI (arrow in C).

Key Facts
- Definition: Intradural ossification associated with chronic post-inflammatory adhesion and clumping of lumbar nerve roots
- Classic imaging appearance
  - Absence of discrete nerve roots in the thecal sac
  - Calcification within
    - Large clump of nerve roots centrally within the thecal sac
    - Soft tissue mass occupying most of the thecal sac
- Other key facts
  - Uncommon entity
  - May be associated with progressive neurologic impairment
  - Small calcified dural plaques are unrelated and asymptomatic

Imaging Findings
<u>General Features</u>
- Best imaging clue: Focal calcific density (CT) or T1 and T2 hyperintensity (fatty marrow) within lumbar nerve root aggregate
<u>CT Myelogram Findings</u>
- Calcifications of the clumped nerve roots or soft tissue mass
  - Thin and linear
  - Masslike and globular
- Intraspinal cysts and loculations
<u>MR Findings</u>
- More subtle than CT
- Linear or globular signal alteration, distinct from nerve root conglomerate
  - Variable signal intensity, hypo- or hyperintense on T1WI and T2WI
  - Hyperintensity represents fatty marrow
  - No post-gadolinium enhancement

Arachnoiditis Ossificans

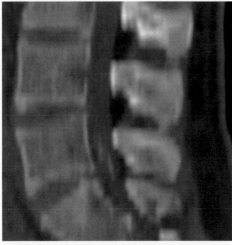

Sagittal reformation of lumbar CT reveals two linear calcifications in the thecal sac, corresponding to the linear hypointensity on MRI.

- Evidence of prior lumbar surgery
- Variable degree of nerve root enhancement

Differential Diagnosis
<u>Retained Pantopaque</u>
- Hyperintense on T1WI and iso- to hypointense on T2WI
- Differentiated from calcification by CT
<u>Spinal Stenosis</u>
- Clumped nerve roots
- Degenerative changes prominent
- No intrathecal calcification
<u>Intrathecal Neoplasm, Carcinomatous Meningitis, Leptomeningeal Spread</u>
- More vigorous enhancement of mass, nerve roots, or focal nodules
- Mass or nodules isointense on T1WI and hyperintense on T2WI

Pathology
<u>General</u>
- Etiology-Pathogenesis
  - In the past, lumbar arachnoiditis more commonly related to trauma or spinal meningitis
    - Tuberculous meningitis
    - Syphilis
  - Now more commonly associated with prior lumbar surgery
    - Especially when multiple or complicated
    - In combination with antecedent multiple or complicated spinal myelography, water or oil based agents
  - Common pathway of
    - Inflammatory cellular reaction
    - Fibrin deposition

Arachnoiditis Ossificans

  - Perineural and leptomeningeal fibrosis
  - Nerve roots adhering to one another and to the thecal sac
 o Ossification results from
 o Ossified intrathecal hematoma
 o Bone fragments from prior trauma or surgery
 o Osseous metaplasia from chronic inflammation and fibrosis
- Epidemiology
 o <1,000 cases of lumbar arachnoiditis reported in the literature over 50 years
 o Arachnoiditis ossificans even rarer
 o Clinical syndrome probably more common

Gross Pathologic-Surgical Features
- Calcified inflammatory, collagenous mass

Microscopic Features
- Fibroblastic proliferation with osseous metaplasia
- Small areas of calcifications

Clinical Issues

Presentation
- No defining clinical symptomatology
- Simulates spinal stenosis and polyneuropathy
- Low back pain
- Radicular or non-radicular leg pain
- Paraparesis
- Bladder and bowel dysfunction

Natural History
- Symptoms usually static, but may fluctuate in severity
- Arachnoiditis ossificans tend to have progressive neurologic deficits compared to lumbar arachnoiditis

Treatment
- Decompressive laminectomy
- Resection of ossified plaques not effective

Prognosis
- Decompressive laminectomy alone may be beneficial

Selected References
1. Frizzell B et al: Arachnoiditis ossificans: MR imaging features in five patients. AJR 177:461-4, 2001
2. Long DM: Chronic adhesive spinal arachnoiditis: pathogenesis, prognosis, and treatment. Neurosurgery Quarterly 2:296-318, 1992

Spinal Cord Multiple Sclerosis

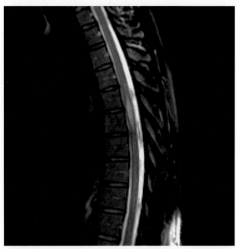

Sagittal T2WI demonstrates a focal intramedullary hyperintense lesion in the thoracic cord.

Key Facts
- Definition: Chronic and relapsing inflammatory and demyelinating disease of the central nervous system with multiple lesions disseminated over time and space
- Classic imaging appearance
  - Peripheral in location
    - Typically in dorsolateral aspect of the cord
  - Less than two vertebral segments in length
  - Less than half the cross-sectional area of the cord
- Other key facts
  - 90% incidence of associated intracranial lesions
  - 10% to 20% isolated spinal cord disease
  - Cervical cord is the most commonly affected spinal cord segment
  - Imaging must be correlated with clinical and laboratory features to confirm the diagnosis

Imaging Findings
General Features
- Best imaging clue: Presence of concomitant intracranial lesions in the periventricular, subcallosal, brain stem, and cerebellar white matter
MR Findings
- Solitary or multifocal lesions
- Peripheral in location, typically dorsal or lateral
- Less than two vertebral segments in length
- Less than half the cross-sectional area of the cord
- Normal or mild focal cord expansion; cord atrophy in late stage
- Isointense or low intensity on T1WI
- High signal intensity on T2WI
- Variable post-gadolinium enhancement
  - Homogeneous or ring enhancement during acute or subacute phase
  - No enhancement during chronic phase

Spinal Cord Multiple Sclerosis

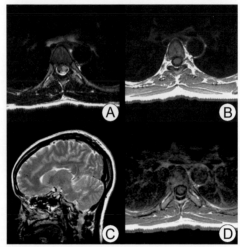

Axial T2WI (A) confirms the eccentrically located intramedullary lesion. Axial T1WI Pre- (B) and post gadolinium (D) demonstrate peripheral enhancement. Sagittal T2 weighted MR through the brain (C) shows a hyperintense lesion involving the corpus callosum.

Imaging Recommendations
- MRI of the brain including high resolution fast spin echo T2 through the corpus callosum
  - Presence of periventricular, subcallosal, brain stem, and cerebellar white matter lesions can help make the diagnosis of multiple sclerosis

Differential Diagnosis
Spinal Cord Ischemia and Infarct
- Sudden onset of symptom
- Posterior columns typically spared in anterior spinal infarct
Idiopathic Transverse Myelitis
- Lesion centrally located
- 3 to 4 segments in length
- Occupying more than two thirds of the cord's cross-sectional area
- No associated intracranial lesions
- Diagnosis of exclusion

Pathology
General
- General Path Comments
  - Focal regions of demyelination of varying size and age scattered throughout the white matter of the CNS
- Genetics
  - Low familial incidence
- Etiology-Pathogenesis
  - Autoimmune, cell-mediated inflammatory process focused on CNS myelin
- Epidemiology
  - Increasing prevalence further north from the equator

Spinal Cord Multiple Sclerosis

- 30 to 80 per 100,000 in Northern US and Europe
- 6 to 14 per 100,000 in Southern US and Europe
- 1 per 100,000 in equatorial regions
  o Adult females more susceptible than males (1.7:1)
  - Men more likely to have the relapsing progressive and chronic progressive forms of spinal cord multiple sclerosis
  - Women more likely to have the relapsing remitting form

Microscopic Features

- Less likely to respect the gray and white matter boundaries compared to intracranial lesions
- Discrete lesions of myelin destruction
- Active lesions full of macrophages
- Chronic lesions gliotic and cavitary
- Perivascular cuffs of lymphocytes and mononuclear cells
- Involvement of the dorsal horns common

Clinical Issues

Presentation
- Principal presenting symptom: Myelopathy, sensory predomination

Natural History
- Onset in third to fourth decades
- Attacks of focal neurologic dysfunction at nonpredictable intervals
  o Lasting weeks
  o Variable recovery
  o 60% of the cases
- Slowly progressive neurologic deterioration
  o Over years
  o Without exacerbations and remissions
  o Less common
- Rapidly progressive neurologic deterioration
  o Death within months
  o Uncommon

Treatment
- IV and oral prednisone
- Immunosuppression therapy
  o Azathioprine
  o Cyclophosphamide
- Supportive therapy
  o Anticholinergics
  o Smooth muscle relaxants

Selected References
1. Tartaglino LM et al: Multiple Sclerosis in the Spinal Cord: MR Appearance and Correlation with Clinical Parameters. Radiology 195:725-32, 1995
2. Campi A et al: Acute Transverse Myelopathy: Spinal and Cranial MR Study with Clinical Follow-up. AJNR 16:115-23, 1995
3. Maravilla KR et al: Magnetic Resonance Demonstration of Multiple Sclerosis Plaques in the Cervical Cord. AJNR 5:685-9, 1984

Spinal Cord Sarcoidosis

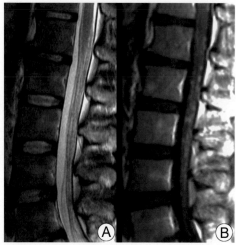

There is suggestion of subtle hyperintense nodules interspersed throughout the cauda equina on sagittal T2WI (A). After intravenous gadolinium, numerous enhancing nodules are clearly evident on sagittal T1WI (B).

Key Facts
- Definition: Chronic, multi-system, noncaseating granulomatous disease of unknown cause
- Classic imaging appearance
  - Protean imaging manifestations, mimicking multiple spinal pathologies
  - Combination of leptomeningeal enhancement with peripherally located intramedullary masslike enhancement suggestive of the disease
- Other key facts
  - Clinical central nervous system involvement in 5% of patients with sarcoidosis
  - At autopsy, 15% of patients with sarcoidosis have central nervous system involvement
  - Isolated neurosarcoidosis in 1.5% of cases
  - Spinal intramedullary sarcoidosis in less than 1% of patients with sarcoidosis
  - Intramedullary lesions most commonly affect the cervical or the upper thoracic cord
  - The diagnosis of intramedullary sarcoidosis may be corroborated by less invasive methods such as angiotensin converting enzyme level, lymph node biopsy, and transbronchial lung biopsy before considering spinal cord biopsy
  - Intraoperative frozen-sections of intramedullary sarcoidosis may be misinterpreted for gliomas

Imaging Findings
MR Findings
- Diffuse cord enlargement
- Cord atrophy in late stages
- Solitary or multiple intramedullary masslike enhancement

Spinal Cord Sarcoidosis

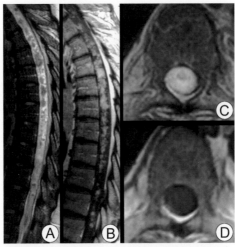

In another patient, sagittal T2WI (A) shows diffuse hyperintensity in the spinal cord, interspersed with nodular isointensities. After intravenous gadolinium, sagittal T1WI (B) reveals patchy and nodular enhancement throughout the spinal cord. Axial T2WI (C) and T1WI (D) demonstrate an enlarged cord.

- o Tendency for peripheral location with broad-based contact with the cord surface
- Leptomeningeal enhancement
- Enhancing nerve roots with or without enhancing nodules
- Regression of findings during therapy, especially leptomeningeal and intramedullary enhancement

Differential Diagnosis
Intramedullary Neoplasm
- Lack of leptomeningeal enhancement
- Enhancement usually involves the whole cross-sectional area of the cord
- The degree of enhancement does not regress significantly after treatment with corticosteroids
Multiple Sclerosis
- Lack of leptomeningeal enhancement
- Presence of intracranial periventricular, subcallosal, brainstem, and cerebellar white matter lesions can help make the diagnosis of multiple sclerosis
Idiopathic Transverse Myelitis
- Lesion centrally located
- 3 to 4 segments in length
- Occupying more than two thirds of the cord's cross-sectional area
- Diagnosis of exclusion

Pathology
General
- General Path Comments
  - o Noncaseating granulomatous inflammation of unknown etiology
- Etiology-Pathogenesis

Spinal Cord Sarcoidosis

- o Leptomeningeal granulomatous inflammation
- o Central spread into the spinal cord through perivascular space
- o Coalescing granulomas forming mass(es)
- o Cord ischemia/infarct secondary to vasculitis
- Epidemiology
  - o Second to fourth decades of life
  - o Sarcoidosis relatively more common in Northern Europeans and African-Americans

Microscopic Features
- Epithelioid and giant cell noncaseating granulomas
- Areas of neural tissue infarction
- Perivascular lymphocytic infiltrate

Clinical Issues
Presentation
- Radiculopathy
- Paraparesis
- Sensory level
- Bladder and bowel dysfunction

Treatment
- Intravenous and/or oral corticosteroids
- Immunosuppressive therapy
  - o Cyclophosphamide
  - o Methotrexate
  - o Cyclosporine

Prognosis
- Favorable response to corticosteroid therapy

Selected References
1. Lexa FJ et al: MR of sarcoidosis in the head and spine: spectrum of manifestations and radiographic response to steroid therapy. AJNR 5:973-82, 1994
2. Junger SS et al: Intramedullary spinal sarcoidosis: clinical and magnetic imaging characteristics. Neurology 43:333-7, 1993
3. Nesbit GM et al: Spinal cord sarcoidosis: A new finding at MR imaging with Gd-DTPA enhancement. Radiology 173:839-43, 1989

Idiopathic Acute Transverse Myelitis

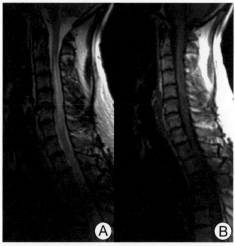

There is an intramedullary lesion in the cervical cord spanning 5 vertebral segments from C2-3 to C7. It is hyperintense on T2WI (A) and hypointense on T1WI (B). There is subtle expansion of the cervical cord at C5 and C6.

Key Facts
- Synonym: Idiopathic acute transverse myelopathy
- Definition
  - Clinical syndrome
  - Monophasic bilateral motor, sensory, and autonomic dysfunction
  - Absence of preexisting neurologic diseases or spinal cord compression
- Classic imaging appearance
  - Central location
  - More than two vertebral segments in length
  - More than two thirds of the cross-sectional area of the cord
- Other key facts
  - Acute onset
  - Thoracic cord most often affected
  - Must exclude other causes of acute transverse myelitis
    - Primary (multiple sclerosis) and secondary (acute disseminated encephalomyelitis) demyelinating diseases
    - Vasculitis such as systemic lupus erythematosus
    - Cord ischemia and infarction
    - Vascular malformations
    - Neoplasm
    - Paraneoplastic myelopathy
    - Complication of radiation therapy

Imaging Findings
General Features
- Best imaging clue: Central holocord lesion more than two vertebral segments in length
MR Findings
- Solitary or multifocal lesions
- Central location

Idiopathic Acute Transverse Myelitis

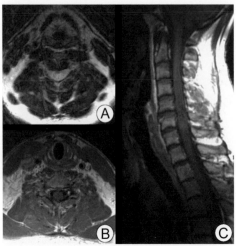

Axial T2WI (A) demonstrates a centrally located intramedullary lesion occupying more than half the cross-sectional area of the cervical cord. After gadolinium, there is no significant enhancement on axial (B) and sagittal (C) T1WI.

- More than two vertebral segments in length
- More than two thirds of the cross-sectional area of the cord
- Normal or mild focal cord expansion; cord atrophy in late stage
- Isointense or low intensity on T1WI
- High signal intensity on T2WI
- Variable post-gadolinium enhancement
  - No enhancement
  - Nodular enhancement
  - Subtle diffuse enhancement
  - Peripheral enhancement
  - Meningeal enhancement
  - More frequent in the subacute than in the acute or chronic stage
  - Resolves over time

Imaging Recommendations
- MRI of the brain including high resolution fast spin echo T2 through the corpus callosum
- To exclude intracranial lesions associated with multiple sclerosis or acute disseminated encephalomyelitis

Differential Diagnosis
Multiple Sclerosis
- Peripheral in location
- Less than two vertebral segments in length
- Less than half the cross-sectional area of the cord
- 90% incidence of associated intracranial lesions
- Relapsing and remitting clinical course

Spinal Cord Neoplasm
- Cord expansion invariably present
- Diffuse or nodular contrast enhancement
- Extensive peri-tumoral edema

Idiopathic Acute Transverse Myelitis

- Associated cystic changes
- Slower clinical progression

Cord Infarct
- Ventral cord location
- Motor signs greater than sensory
- Immediate onset (minutes, rather than hours, days)
- Less mass effect initially

Pathology
General
- Etiology-Pathogenesis
  - Possible association with previous viral infection or vaccination in some cases
  - Autoimmune phenomenon with formation of antigen-antibody complexes
  - Small vessel vasculopathy resulting in cord ischemia
  - Associated demyelination process
- Epidemiology
  - Majority of the cases occurred in late winter through spring in one series

Microscopic Features
- Nonspecific necrosis of gray and white matter
- Demyelination
- Perivascular lymphocytic infiltrate

Clinical Issues
Presentation
- Prodrome of generalized body aches
- Rapid progression to maximal neurologic deficits within days
- Bilateral sensory and motor deficits
- Urinary bladder involvement common

Treatment
- High-dose intravenous steroid pulse therapy

Prognosis
- One third of patients experience good recovery
- One third mild recovery
- One third poor recovery with persistent complete deficits

Selected References
1. Choi KH et al: Idiopathic Transverse Myelitis: MR Characteristics. AJNR 17:1151-60, 1996
2. Tartaglino LM et al: Idiopathic Acute Transverse Myelitis: MR Imaging Findings. Radiology 201:661-9, 1996
3. Campi A et al: Acute Transverse Myelopathy: Spinal and Cranial MR Study with Clinical Follow-up. AJNR 16:115-23, 1995

CIDP

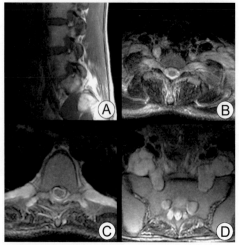

Sagittal T1WI (A) shows diffuse hypointense enlargement of the nerve roots and lumbar plexus. Axial T2WI through the cervical (B), thoracic (C), and lumbar levels (D) show diffuse nerve hyperintensity and plexus enlargement.

Key Facts
- Synonym(s): Chronic Inflammatory Demyelinating Polyneuropathy
- Definition: Chronic demyelinating neuropathy
- Classic imaging appearance: Diffuse T2 hyperintense plexus and peripheral nerve enlargement
- May be either idiopathic or secondary to infection, neoplasm, or connective tissue disease
- Possible association with concurrent CNS demyelination
  - CNS disease is frequently subclinical

Imaging Findings
General Features
- Best imaging clue: Diffuse bilateral peripheral nerve enlargement
CT Findings
- Diffuse enlargement of the cauda equina, nerve roots/plexuses, and proximal nerves
MR Findings
- T1WI: Marked enlargement of the cauda equina, nerve roots/plexuses, and proximal nerves with contrast enhancement
- T2WI: Abnormal hyperintensity
Other Modality Findings
- Ultrasound: Diffuse hypoechoic nerve enlargement
Imaging Recommendations
- Use surface coil if possible
- T2 and enhanced T1 coronal and axial imaging sequences with fat suppression best delineate extent and location of abnormalities
- Consider brain MRI to detect subclinical CNS demyelination

CIDP

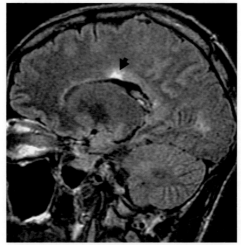

Sagittal FLAIR brain image shows a typical paraventricular demyelinating lesion (arrow) of the corpus callosum along the callosal-septal interface

Differential Diagnosis
Guillain-Barre (AIDP)
- Distinguished by duration of onset and typical clinical course of ascending paralysis with sensation relatively preserved

Inherited Demyelinating Neuropathy (Charcot-Marie-Tooth, Dejerine-Sottas Disease)
- Genetic testing and clinical phenotype help distinguish from CIDP

Neurofibromatosis Type 1
- Genetic testing and distinctive clinical stigmata help distinguish from CIDP

Pathology
General
- General Path Comments
  - Multifocal demyelination affecting primarily the spinal roots/nerves, plexuses, and proximal nerve trunks
  - May extend more distally
- Etiology-Pathogenesis
  - Idiopathic
  - Secondary to infectious, neoplastic, or collagen-vascular disease

Gross Pathologic-Surgical Features
- Extensive nerve enlargement

Microscopic Features
- Enlarged nerves with onion-bulb formations
- Nerve demyelination and remyelination

Clinical Issues
Presentation
- Mixed sensorimotor neuropathy
- Either motor or sensory symptoms may predominate
- May be idiopathic or associated with HIV, Lyme disease, connective tissue diseases, or lymphoma and other malignancies

- Some patients have concurrent CNS demyelination (usually subclinical)

Natural History

- May show chronic progressive, step-wise progressive, or recurrent behavior

Treatment

- Immunomodulation or immunosuppression therapy
- Prednisolone therapy, plasmapheresis, or intravenous immunoglobulin (IVIG)

Prognosis

- Average disease duration is 7.5 years
- Mildly affected patients tend to recover; severely affected patients are more likely to have chronic symptoms or mortality related to CIDP

Selected References
1. Cros D: Peripheral Neuropathy. First ed. Philadelphia: Lippincott Williams & Wilkins: 432, 2001
2. Van den Bergh PY et al: Chronic demyelinating hypertrophic brachial plexus neuropathy. Muscle nerve 23(2): 283-8, 2000
3. Mizuno K et al: Chronic inflammatory demyelinating polyradiculoneuropathy with diffuse and massive peripheral nerve hypertrophy: distinctive clinical and magnetic resonance imaging features. Muscle nerve 21(6);805-8, 1998

Vitamin B12 Deficiency

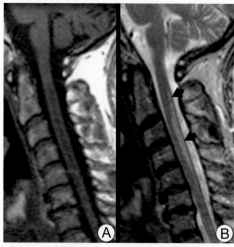

Vitamin B12 deficiency: (A) Sagittal T1WI of the cervical spine demonstrates mild cord enlargement and hypointensity within the dorsal columns. (B) Sagittal T2WI confirms hyperintensity within the dorsal columns (arrows), sparing the remainder of the cord.

Key Facts
- Synonym(s): Subacute combined degeneration, combined system disease
- Definition: Vitamin B12 deficiency produces selective degeneration of dorsal and lateral columns
- Classic imaging appearance: Mild cord enlargement with abnormal signal within the dorsal and/or lateral columns
- Vitamin B12 is found in low concentrations in meat but not in vegetables
- B12 deficiency may be identified in either adults or infants
  - Most adult cases (in the US) arise in context of pernicious anemia
  - Rarely in infants of strict vegetarian mothers or Vegan adolescents
  - Symptoms arise from demyelination

Imaging Findings
General Features
- Best imaging clue: Characteristic T2 hyperintensity confined to dorsal spinal cord columns
- Rarely extramedullary hematopoesis in severe cases of anemia
CT Findings
- Spine: Difficult or impossible to diagnose on CT
- Brain: No specific findings in adults; in infants may see severe atrophy that improves following parenteral B12 therapy
MR Findings
- T1WI: Mild spinal cord enlargement and hypointensity in the dorsal cord; does not enhance
- T2WI: Hyperintensity distributed along same topography
Imaging Recommendations
- Sagittal T2WI clearly defines predilection for dorsal columns
  - Axial T2WI confirms localization

Vitamin B12 Deficiency

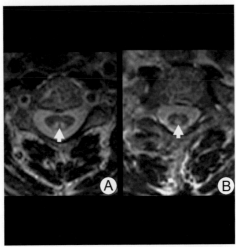

Vitamin B12 deficiency. (A, B) Axial T2WIs confirm abnormal hyperintensity is located within the dorsal columns only (arrows). The lateral columns are normal.

Differential Diagnosis
<u>Amyotrophic Lateral Sclerosis (ALS)</u>
- Specifically involves the corticospinal tracts and anterior horn motor cells
  - Ventral spinal cord atrophy with T2 hyperintensity
  - May extend rostrally into centrum semiovale/ subcortical white matter
- Spares the dorsal columns
- Characteristic clinical presentation and disease course is readily distinguished from B12 deficiency

<u>Inflammatory Demyelination</u>
- Multiple sclerosis or acute disseminated encephalomyelitis (ADEM)
- Have characteristic clinical presentations
- Focal lesions do not show specificity for lateral or dorsal columns

<u>Transverse Myelitis</u>
- Acute presentation
- Diffuse multisegmental cord signal change with swelling

<u>Cord Infarction</u>
- Hyperacute presentation, predominantly ventral cord changes, and motor > sensory symptoms

Pathology
<u>General</u>
- General Path Comments
  - Primary finding is selective dorsolateral spinal cord degeneration
  - Peripheral nerves frequently involved as well
- Etiology-Pathogenesis
  - Most common etiology (in US) is pernicious anemia
    - Antibodies to intrinsic factor (IF) and gastric parietal cells prevent normal secretion of IF
    - Absence of IF prevents normal absorption of vitamin B12 in the terminal ileum

Vitamin B12 Deficiency

- o Other etiologies include fish tapeworm (D. latum) infestation, Crohn's disease, celiac disease, bacterial overgrowth in intestinal blind loops, and strict vegetarian diet
- o Folate deficiency produces similar clinical findings to B12 deficiency
- Epidemiology
  - o Pernicious anemia is more common in Scandinavian and "English speaking" populations, but found within all racial groups
  - o Males affected slightly more common than females
  - o Diagnosis usually in fifth to eighth decade

Gross Pathologic-Surgical Features
- CNS lesions found in three quarters of fulminant cases
  - o Gray discoloration of the posterior and lateral columns at autopsy
  - o Most severe in middle and upper thoracic cord
  - o Patchy demyelination may be found in cerebral white matter

Microscopic Features
- Myelin sheath degeneration; axonal degeneration to a lesser extent

Clinical Issues
Presentation
- Frequently insidious symptom onset
  - o Spinal cord symptoms include motor (spastic paraparesis, gait unsteadiness) and sensory findings (parasthesias, absent reflexes, loss of joint position sense and vibration sense)
  - o Mental status decline with progressive psychomotor regression (confusion, depression, delusions, mental slowness)
- Laboratory abnormalities
  - o Macrocytic anemia (MCV > 100)
  - o Diminished plasma B12 level

Treatment
- Treatment arrests degenerative process but will not restore destroyed nerve fibers
- Cornerstones of therapy
  - o Life-long parenteral B12 administration
  - o Address treatable causes

Prognosis
- Spontaneous improvement without treatment uncommon
- May see dramatic clinical improvement following B12 therapy

Selected References
1.   Locatelli ER et al: MRI in vitamin B12 deficiency myelopathy. Can J Neurol Sci 26(1): 60-3, 1999
2.   Taybi H et al: Radiology of syndromes, metabolic disorders, and skeletal dysplasias. Fourth ed. St. Louis: Mosby-Yearbook Publishing, 1996
3.   Rowland L: Merritt's Textbook of Neurology. Eighth ed. Lea & Febiger: Philadelphia, 1989

NEOPLASMS

Spinal Osteoid Osteoma

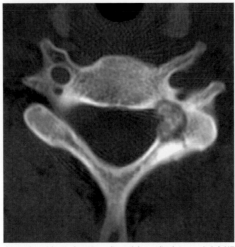

A 12-year-old male with neck pain relieved by salicylates. Axial NECT shows a discrete lucent mass with a calcified nidus in the left pedicle of the C6 vertebra. Note the surrounding reactive sclerosis and small size (<1.5 cm), characteristic for osteoid osteoma.

Key Facts
- Definition: Benign osteoblastic tumor with central core of vascular osteoid tissue, peripheral sclerosis
- Osteoid osteoma (OO) = tumor of children, young adults
- 10% in spine (most common cause of painful scoliosis in adolescents)
- Classic presentation = night pain relieved by salicylates/NSAIDS
- Imaging findings: <1.5 cm round low density + surrounding sclerosis

Imaging Findings
General Features
- Best imaging clue: Hypodense nidus with Ca++, surrounding sclerosis
- Neural arch >> vertebral body
CT Findings
- NECT
  - Lesion <1.5 cm (larger = osteoblastoma)
  - Well-defined low density nidus
    - +/- Ca++
  - Variable surrounding sclerosis
- CECT: Variable enhancement
MR Findings
- T1WI: Hypo- > isointense (compared to marrow)
- T2WI
  - Hyperintense > intermediate signal
    - Variable Ca++ (very hypointense)
    - Surrounding hyperintensity may reflect inflammation
- Variable enhancement (minimal to intense)
Other Modality Findings
- Radiography
  - Classic
    - Discrete round/oval nidus with surrounding sclerosis

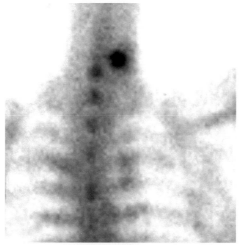

Same case as previous page. Radionuclide bone scan shows a solitary focus of marked radiotracer accumulation within the nidus in the lower left cervical spine. The history and this finding in a young patient is very suggestive for osteoid osteoma (case courtesy of J. Crim).

- Lesion at/near apex (concave aspect) of scoliotic curve
  - Common: Normal, subtle sclerosis, sometimes only scoliosis
- Radionuclide scan
  - Nidus shows marked radiotracer accumulation
  - "Double density sign" = small central high uptake (nidus) with surrounding less intense zone of uptake (osseous reaction)

Imaging Recommendations
- Radionuclide scan + NECT
- MR if radiculopathy or myelopathy

Differential Diagnosis

Osteoblastoma
- Larger (>1.5 cm)
- Expansile lesion of neural arch/pedicle
- Neurologic deficits more common

Sclerotic Metastasis, Lymphoma
- Older patients
- Often involves pedicle, destroys posterior body cortex
- Associated soft-tissue mass common

Aneurysmal Bone Cyst
- Larger, expansile
- Often multicystic with hemorrhagic fluid-fluid levels

Benign (Nonneoplastic) Reactive Sclerosis
- Facet sclerosis (spondylolysis; contralateral to absent pedicle)
- Unusual/chronic infection (rare)

Spinal Osteoid Osteoma

Pathology

<u>General</u>
- General Path Comments
  - Location
    - Femur > tibia > hands/feet > vertebral
    - Lumbar > cervical > thoracic > sacrum
    - Posterior element (lamina, facet, pedicle)
    - Vertebral body < 10%
- Epidemiology
  - 12% of all benign skeletal neoplasms
  - 10% in axial skeleton
  - 59% lumbar, 27% cervical, 12% thoracic, 2% sacrum
  - Majority of patients between 10-20 years
  - M: F = 2-3:1

<u>Gross Pathologic-Surgical Features</u>
- Sharply-demarcated, round, pink-red mass (nidus)

<u>Microscopic Features</u>
- Nidus: Well-organized interconnecting trabecular bone in various stages of maturity within a highly vascular fibrous connective tissue stroma
- Similar to osteoblastoma
- No malignant degeneration

Clinical Issues

<u>Presentation</u>
- Night pain with relief from salicylates/NSAIDS
- Symptoms: Painful scoliosis, focal/radicular pain, gait disturbance, muscle atrophy
- Scoliosis (70%) related to muscle spasm
- In pediatric patients, torticollis, spinal stiffness, scoliosis may occur

<u>Natural History</u>
- Surgical resection is curative in most cases
- Spontaneous healing has been reported

<u>Treatment</u>
- Complete excision
  - New: CT-guided percutaneous excision
  - Thermo-/photocoagulation
- Conservative observation (patients with well controlled symptoms)

<u>Prognosis</u>
- Recurrence extremely rare after surgical excision

Selected References
1. Cove JA et al: Osteoid osteoma of the spine treated with percutaneous computed tomography-guided thermocoagulation. Spine 25:1283-6, 2000
2. Murphey MD et al: Primary tumors of the spine: Radiologic-pathologic correlation. Radiographics 16: 1131-58, 1996
3. Kransdorf MJ et al: Osteoid osteoma. Radiographics 11:671-96, 1991

Spinal Osteoblastoma

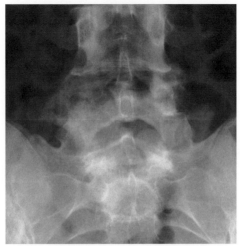

A 15-year-old male presented with dull right-sided low back pain. Anteroposterior radiograph of the lumbosacral spine shows an expansile mass replacing the right L5 pedicle. The posterior neural arch appears intact. The right vertebral body cortex is indistinct.

Key Facts
- Definition: Vascular, osteoid and bone-forming tumor
- 40% of osteoblastomas (OBs) occur in the spine
- 80% of patients < 30y
- Pathology similar to osteoid osteoma (OO) but OB > 1.5-2 cm
- Causes dull, localized pain, neurologic symptoms > OO

Imaging Findings
General Features
- Best imaging clue: Expansile lesion of neural arch/pedicle
CT Findings
- NECT: 3 patterns
  - Most common
    - Bone remodeled by well-circumscribed, lucent, expansile lesion
    - Matrix mineralization (multifocal small Ca++)
    - Sclerotic rim
  - Central radiolucent area +/- Ca++, surrounding sclerosis (like OO but > 1.5cm diameter)
  - Aggressive OB (bone destruction, soft-tissue infiltration, variable Ca++)
- CECT: +/- enhancement
MR Findings
- T1WI
  - Low/intermediate signal
- T2WI
  - Intermediate/high-signal intensity
  - Extensive peritumoral edema common
  - May have large soft-tissue component
  - May extend into vertebral body

Spinal Osteoblastoma

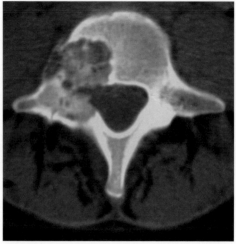

Same case as previous page. Axial NECT shows the well-demarcated expansile lesion has a "ground glass" appearance. Minimal cortical destruction with extension into the right lateral recess is present. Lesion centered in the pedicle, size > 1.5 cm is typical for osteoblastoma (case courtesy J. Crim).

Other Modality Findings
- Radiography
  - Expansile "ground glass" lesion
  - 50% have scoliosis (lesion is at apex of concave curve)
- Radionuclide scans show intense uptake
- Angiography = vascular (intense, prolonged contrast accumulation)

Imaging Recommendations
- NECT for bone detail
- MR for soft tissue extent, effect on cord/roots

Differential Diagnosis (Varies with Pattern)

Osteoid Osteoma
- Smaller (<1.5 cm)
- Stable size vs. slow growth for OB

Aneurysmal Bone Cyst (ABC)
- ABC component present in 10%-15% of OBs
- Multiple blood-filled cavities with fluid-fluid levels
- May involve contiguous vertebrae (rare with OB)

Metastasis
- Older patients

Other Primary Bone Tumors
- Osteosarcoma
  - Rare in spine
  - Periosteal new bone
  - Prominent soft-tissue component
- Cartilage tumor
  - Enchondroma, osteochondroma
  - Punctate or "popcorn-like" Ca++

Spinal Osteoblastoma

- Giant cell tumor
  - Patients usually 20-40y
  - Vertebral body > posterior elements
  - Rarely occurs above sacrum

Nonneoplastic Mimics
- Fibrous dysplasia
  - Polyostotic involvement common (OB almost never multiple)
- Langerhans cell histiocytosis
  - Vertebral body (often causes vertebra plana)
  - Less expansile

Pathology
General
- General Path Comments
  - Lesion > 1.5cm (smaller classified as OOs)
- Epidemiology
  - 90% diagnosed in 2nd, 3rd decades of life
  - M: F = 2-2.5:1
  - 40% cervical, 25% lumbar, 20% thoracic, 15-20% sacrum

Gross Pathologic-Surgical Features
- Usually well circumscribed, surrounded by shell of cortical bone/ periosteum
- Friable, highly vascular tumor

Microscopic Features
- Similar to OO (greater osteoid production, vascularity)
  - Interconnecting trabecular bone + fibrovascular stroma
  - Numerous osteoclasts (multinucleated giant cells)
- ABC-like component found in 10-15%
- "Aggressive" OBs (like osteosarcoma, contain epithelioid osteoblasts)

Clinical Issues
Presentation
- Scoliosis, dull localized pain +/- neurologic symptoms

Natural History
- Grow slowly

Treatment
- Surgical resection +/- preoperative embolization

Prognosis
- 10-15% recurrence (50% for aggressive OBs)

Selected References
1. Murphey MD et al: Primary tumors of the spine: Radiologic-pathologic correlation. RadioGraphics 16: 1131-58, 1996
2. Boriani S et al: Osteoblastoma of the spine. Clin Ortho Rel Res 278: 37-45, 1992
3. Nemoto O et al: Osteoblastoma of the spine. Spine 15: 1272-80, 1990

Spinal Osteochondroma

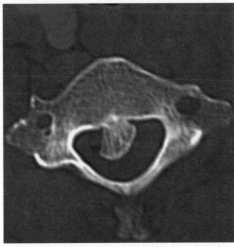

A 25-year-old male with myelopathy. Axial NECT shows a pedunculated bony projection extending into the spinal canal. Note continuity between marrow, cortex of the osseous excrescence with normal underlying bone, typical for osteochondroma.

Key Facts
- Synonym: Osteocartilaginous exostosis; exostosis
- Definition: Cartilage-covered osseous excrescence
- Most common benign bone lesion
  - 30%-45% of all benign bone tumors
  - Spine = < 5% of osteochondromas (OCs)
  - Peak age = 10-30y
- Classic imaging appearance: Sessile "cauliflower" appearance with continuity between marrow and cortex of lesion to underlying bone
- Rapid growth suggests malignant transformation to chondrosarcoma

Imaging Findings
General Features
- Best imaging clue: Continuity of marrow and cortex with underlying bone
- Develops in bones that form through endochondral ossification (physis)
CT Findings
- NECT
  - Sessile or pedunculated bony projection
  - Cortex of parent bone flares into cortex of OC
  - Cartilaginous cap may contain Ca++
MR Findings
- T1WI
  - Hyperintense signal centrally (yellow marrow)
  - Hypointense cortex
  - Hyaline cartilage cap (often small, hypo-/isointense)
- T2WI
  - Isointense signal centrally (yellow marrow)
  - Hypointense cortex
  - Hyaline cartilage cap hyperintense

Spinal Osteochondroma

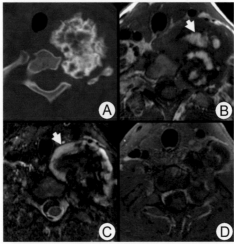

A 20-year-old female with hereditary multiple exostoses. Axial CT (A) shows "cauliflower" osteochondroma. (B) Axial T1WI shows central hyperintense marrow (arrow), hypointense cortex. Axial STIR image (C) shows a hyperintense cartilage cap (arrow). Post-contrast T1WI (D) demonstrates peripheral enhancement.

- o In adults, if cartilage cap >1.5 cm raises concern of malignant transformation (chondrosarcoma)
- Contrast-enhanced T1WI: Peripheral enhancement described

<u>Other Modality Findings</u>
- Radiography
  - o Sessile/pedunculated osseous protuberance
  - o Flaring of parent bone cortex at OC attachment
  - o Small lesions may be difficult to detect (15% normal)

<u>Imaging Recommendations</u>
- NECT for bone detail
- MRI for evaluation of spinal cord, nerves

Differential Diagnosis
<u>Chondrosarcoma</u>
- Lytic destructive lesion with sclerotic margins, +/- soft tissue mass
- Chondroid matrix (rings and arcs)
- May arise from malignant degeneration of OC (thick cartilaginous cap)

<u>Osteoblastoma</u>
- Expansile lesion of neural arch/pedicle

<u>Aneurysmal Bone Cyst</u>
- Expansile, multicystic; fluid-fluid levels

Pathology
<u>General</u>
- General Path Comments
  - o Location: <5% vertebra (85% metaphysis of long tubular bone)
    - Cervical spine (50%; predilection for C2)
    - Thoracic > Lumbar >> Sacrum
    - Posterior elements (spinous/transverse process) > vertebral body

- o Cartilaginous cap thickness correlates with age of patient
- Genetics
  - o Sporadic: None known
  - o Hereditary multiple exostoses (HME)
    - Autosomal dominant
    - Variable expression
- Etiology-Pathogenesis
  - o Arises during development when epiphyseal cartilage is trapped outside the physeal plate; grows at its tip as cartilage ossifies
  - o May be radiation induced (dose-dependent)
    - Occurs at periphery of XRT treatment field
    - Typically in patients < 2 years at time of XRT
- Epidemiology
  - o OCs = 30-45% of all benign bone tumors
  - o <5% of OCs occur in spine
  - o 7-9% of patients with multiple hereditary OCs have spine lesion
  - o Male predominance in solitary form (1.5-2.5:1)

Gross Pathologic-Surgical Features
- Bony excrescence with cartilaginous cap; cortex and medullary cavity contiguous with parent bone

Microscopic Features
- Similar to normal bone
- Mature cancellous, cortical, and cartilaginous elements

Clinical Issues
Presentation
- Painless, slowly growing mass typical
- Mean age 30y in solitary, 22y in multiple exostoses
- Myelopathy can occur (onset often after trauma)
  - o 34% of patients with solitary OC, 77% of patients with multiple OCs
- Palpable mass in lesions that protrude posteriorly
- Dysphagia, hoarseness, pharyngeal mass can occur with anterior lesions

Natural History
- Complications: Fracture, irritation/damage to nerves, vessels, spinal cord
- Malignant transformation 1-5% solitary lesions; 3-5% multiple lesions
- Spontaneous resolution has been described in children & adolescents
- Growth usually stops at puberty
- Surgical resection is curative in most cases
- Markers for malignant degeneration
  - o Growth after skeletal maturity
  - o Increased cartilage cap (> 1.5 cm in adults)

Treatment
- Surgical excision
- Conservative management in asymptomatic patients

Prognosis
- Recurrence rare, but can occur if incomplete excision
- 89% improvement in symptoms after surgery

Selected References
1. Murphey MD et al: Imaging of osteochondroma: Variants and complications with radiologic-pathologic correlation. RadioGraphics 20:1407-34, 2000
2. Morikawa M et al: Osteochondroma of the cervical spine: MR findings. Clin Imaging 19: 275-8, 1995
3. Albrecht S et al: On spinal osteochondromas. J Neurosurg 77: 247-52, 1992

Vertebral Hemangioma

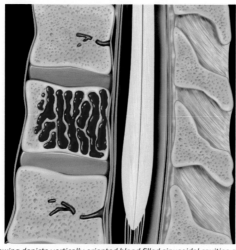

Sagittal drawing depicts vertically oriented blood filled sinusoidal cavities characteristic of hemangioma. The lesion is entirely confined to the vertebral body, typical of benign hemangiomas

Key Facts
- Synonym(s): None
- Definition: Benign vertebral body vascular tumor
- Classic imaging appearance: Hypodense lesion (CT) with coarse, vertically-oriented trabeculae; hyperintense (MRI) on both T1WI and T2WI
- Most common spinal axis tumor
  - Incidental lesion identified on imaging performed for unrelated reasons
  - Rarer presentation (clinical or radiographic) is "aggressive hemangioma"
    - Radiographic diagnostic criteria are lesion growth, bone destruction, vertebral collapse, absence of fat in lesion, and active vascular component
    - May extend epidurally and cause cord compression

Imaging Findings
General Features
- Best imaging clue: Well-circumscribed, hypodense lesion with coarse vertical trabeculae ("white polka dots") on axial CT
CT Findings
- Hypodense lesion centered in vertebral body
  - Sparse, thickened trabeculae surrounded by hypodense fat
  - "Spotted" appearance on axial images
  - Aggressive lesions show avid contrast enhancement
MR Findings
- Typical "benign" (fatty stroma) hemangioma
  - T1WI – hyperintense, with avid contrast enhancement
  - T2WI – hyperintense
  - Occasional radiographically benign lesions are isointense or hypointense on T1WI, and difficult to distinguish from metastases

Vertebral Hemangioma

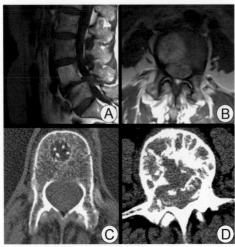

Typical (benign) hemangioma: (A, B) T1WIs show a hyperintense L4 vertebral lesion without epidural expansion. (C) Typical CT appearance (different patient) of well-circumscribed lesion with sparse, thickened trabeculae. Aggressive hemangiom:a (D) Axial CT shows destructive expansion into the epidural space.

- "Aggressive" ("malignant") hemangioma
  - T1WI – isointense to hypointense, with avid contrast enhancement
  - T2WI – hyperintense
  - Pathologic fracture or epidural extension common
  - Clinically aggressive hemangiomas are usually radiographically aggressive as well

Other Modality Findings
- Plain film: Vertebral body lesion with coarse vertical trabeculae resembling corduroy
- Angiography: Normal to hypervascular stain; aggressive lesions stain vividly

Imaging Recommendations
- Both CT and MR can permit a specific diagnosis
  - MR best demonstrates aggressive characteristics
    - Sagittal and axial T1WI images most useful to characterize composition
    - Axial T2WI and enhanced T1WI best for characterizing epidural extent and cord compromise (aggressive lesions)
  - Axial bone algorithm CT is most useful for characteristic features that distinguish hemangioma from metastatic lesion
- Angiography unnecessary unless embolization is being considered

Differential Diagnosis
Vertebral Metastases
- Characteristically extends into pedicles
- Hypointense on T1WI, hypointense to hyperintense (to marrow) on T2WI
- T1WI sequence helps distinguish from benign hemangioma
- May be difficult to distinguish from "vascular" or "aggressive" hemangioma; consider CT

Vertebral Hemangioma

Focal Fatty Marrow
- Incidental rounded focus of marrow fat that is conspicuous on MR imaging
- STIR sequence will show marked lesion hypointensity; hemangiomas typically retain some high signal due to vascular components

Pathology
General
- General Path Comments
  - Slow growing
  - Capillary, cavernous, or venous origin
    - Cavernous hemangiomas most common
- Epidemiology
  - Common – 10-12% of adult population
  - 25-30% multiple; particularly in thoracic spine
  - Peak incidence fourth to sixth decades
  - Benign lesions M = F; aggressive lesions slightly more common in women

Gross Pathologic-Surgical Features
- Vast majority confined to vertebral body proper
  - May be small or occupy entire vertebral body
  - Uncommonly involve posterior elements/pedicles (10-15%)
- Thoracic lesions are more often aggressive than at other locations

Microscopic Features
- Benign lesions show mature, thin-walled, endothelium-lined capillary and cavernous sinuses interspersed among sparse, osseous trabeculae and fatty stromata
- Aggressive lesions contain less fat and more vascular stromata

Clinical Issues
Presentation
- Benign hemangiomas are incidentally discovered
- Symptomatic (aggressive) hemangiomas present with intense, localized spinal pain, myelopathy and/or radiculopathy from osseous expansion, pathologic fracture, and/or epidural extension

Treatment
- Benign (fatty) hemangiomas – no treatment necessary
- Aggressive hemangiomas – first-line therapy is vertebroplasty in conjunction with embolization and surgery as needed

Prognosis
- Benign (fatty) hemangiomas – incidental lesions, excellent prognosis
- Aggressive vascular hemangiomas – variable depending on size of lesion, degree of epidural extension, and presence/absence of cord compression

Selected References
1. Baudrez VC et al: Benign vertebral hemangioma: MR-histological correlation. Skeletal Radiol 30(8): 442-6, 2001
2. Cross JJ et al: Imaging of compressive vertebral hemangiomas. Eur Radiol 10(6): 997-1002, 2000
3. Pastushyn AI et al: Vertebral hemangiomas: diagnosis, management, natural history and clinicopathological correlates in 86 patients. Surg Neurol 50(6): 535-47, 1998

Chordoma

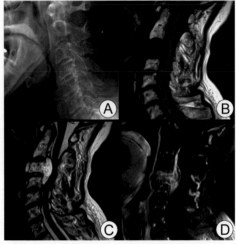

Lateral plain film (A) in a patient with neck pain appears normal. Sagittal pre-contrast T1-, T2-, and post-contrast T1W1 (B, C, D) show diffuse marrow replacement with epidural mass, cord compression. The T2 hyperintensity and heterogeneous enhancement are typical for vertebral chordoma.

Key Facts
- Definition: Malignant tumor arising from notochord remnants
- Midline lobular soft-tissue mass with osseous destruction
- Sacrococcygeal > Spheno-occipital >> Vertebral body
- 2-4% of primary malignant bone tumors
- Histologic identification of physaliphorous cell confirms diagnosis

Imaging Findings
General Features
- Best imaging clue: Mass is hyperintense to discs on T2WI
- Heterogeneous destructive mass of sacrum or vertebral body
  - May extend into disc, involve 2 adjacent vertebrae
  - May extend into epidural/perivertebral space, compress cord
  - May extend along nerve roots, enlarge neural foramina
CT Findings
- NECT
  - Destructive, lytic lesion
  - Most have associated hypodense soft tissue mass
  - Sclerosis in 40-60%
  - Amorphous intratumoral Ca++
    - Sacrum > 70%
    - Vertebra 30%
- CECT
  - Mild/moderate enhancement
  - +/- inhomogeneous areas (cystic necrosis)
MR Findings
- T1WI
  - Heterogeneous hypo- to isointense (compared to marrow)
- T2WI
  - Hyperintense to CSF, intervertebral discs

Chordoma

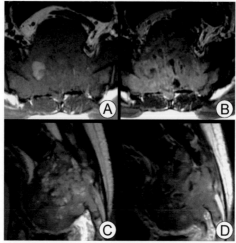

Axial pre- and post-contrast T1WI (A, B) show a destructive, enhancing sacral mass. Sagittal T2WI (C) and post-contrast T1WI (D) show mixed signal throughout the mass. Chordoma was found at surgery. Many chordomas are very hyperintense on T2WI.

   o May have low signal septations (fibrous)
- Variable enhancement – blush to intense enhancement

Other Modality Findings
- Plain films: Lucent lesion with sclerosis
- Bone scan: "cold" lesion

Imaging Recommendations
- MR for soft tissue (STIR/fat-saturated T2WI, contrast-enhanced T1WI)
- NECT for bone detail

Differential Diagnosis

Chondrosarcoma
- Neural arch > vertebral body
- Chondroid matrix (rings and arcs)
- Similar MR characteristics

Giant Cell Tumor
- Heterogeneous MR signal with blood products, low T2 signal

Metastases / Multiple Myeloma / Lymphoma
- Multifocal disease; heterogeneous T2 signal

Sacrococcygeal Teratoma
- Heterogeneous MR signal (fat – T1 hyperintense)
- Pediatric patients

Ecchordosis Physaliphora (rare)
- Benign, nonneoplastic ectopic notochordal remnant(s)
- Usually at skull base but can occur anywhere (including intradural)

Pathology

General
- General Path Comments
  - Location

Chordoma

- Sacrococcygeal 50%; spheno-occipital 35%; vertebral body 15%
- Vertebral body: Cervical (20-50%) > lumbar > thoracic
- Embryology-Anatomy
  - Tumor arises from notochordal remnants
    - Notochord (column of cells ventral to neural tube) arises 3rd gestational week, disappears by 7th week
    - Rests of notochord cells occur in axial skeleton from coccyx to dorsum sellae
- Etiology-Pathogenesis
  - Arises from notochord remnants
- Epidemiology
  - 2-4% of primary malignant bone neoplasms
  - Peak incidence 5th – 6th decades (rare in children)
  - M: F = 2:1 spine (no gender predilection in sacral chordoma)

Gross Pathologic-Surgical Features
- Lobulated, soft, greyish gelatinous mass

Microscopic Features
- 3 types described
  - Typical: Lobules, sheets, and cords of clear cells with intracytoplasmic vacuoles (physaliphorous cells); abundant mucin
  - Chondroid: Hyaline cartilage (usually spheno-occipital region)
  - Dedifferentiated: Sarcomatous elements (rare, highly malignant)
- Immunohistochemistry: + cytokeratin, + epithelial membrane antigen

Clinical Issues
Presentation
- Location dependent: Pain, numbness, weakness, incontinence

Natural History
- Slow-growing
- Distant metastases 5-40% (lung, liver, lymph nodes, bone)

Treatment
- Surgical resection with adjuvant XRT
- Local recurrence common

Prognosis
- Poor prognostic factors
  - Large size
  - Subtotal resection, local recurrence
  - Microscopic necrosis
  - Ki-67 index >5%
- 5 year survival up to 84%

Selected References
1. Bergh P et al: Prognostic factors in chordoma of the sacrum and mobile spine: a study of 39 patients. Cancer 88:2122-34, 2000
2. Wippold FJ et al: Clinical and imaging features of cervical chordoma. AJR 172:1423-6, 1999
3. Murphey MD et al: Primary tumors of the spine: Radiologic-pathologic correlation. RadioGraphics 16:1131-58, 1996

Spinal Plasmacytoma

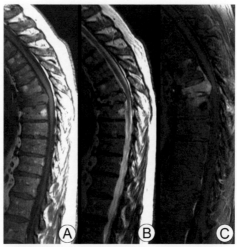

Sagittal pre-contrast T1WI (A), T2WI (B) show an upper thoracic spine compression fracture with kyphosis, moderate cord compression. The adjacent discs are spared. (C) Post-contrasted fat-saturated T1WI demonstrates uniform enhancement extending into the epidural space. Plasmacytoma.

Key Facts
- Definition: Solitary plasma cell tumor of bone (SBP) or soft tissue
- May represent early (Stage I) multiple myeloma (MM)
- Vertebral body = Most common site of SBP
- Classic imaging appearance = Hypointense vertebra (T1WI) with cortical "infoldings," curvilinear low-signal areas

Imaging Findings
General Features
- Best imaging clue: Hypointense marrow with low-signal, curvilinear areas
- Caution: Must exclude **second** unanticipated lesion (33% of cases)
CT Findings
- NECT
  - Common
    - Lytic, destructive vertebral body lesion
    - Compression fracture +/- associated soft- tissue mass
  - Uncommon: Osteosclerosis (3%)
  - Rare: Involvement of intervertebral disc, adjacent vertebrae (if present, helpful differentiating feature from metastasis)
- CECT: Usually little/no detectable enhancement
MR Findings
- T1WI
  - Solitary vertebral body lesion
    - Marrow iso/hypointense (compared to muscle)
    - Contains curvilinear low-signal areas and/or cortical irregularities ("infoldings" caused by endplate fxs)
    - Variable degrees of compression
    - Posterior elements involved in most cases
    - +/- associated soft-tissue mass (paraspinous or epidural with "draped curtain" sign)

Spinal Plasmacytoma

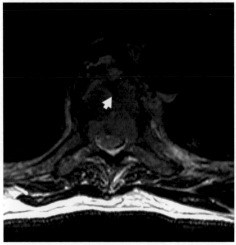

Same case as previous page. Axial T1WI shows marrow replacement, destruction of posterior vertebral body cortex and moderate canal narrowing. (Arrow) indicates "infolded" cortical bone.

- o Scanning entire spine reveals second lesion in 1/3 of cases
- T2WI
  - o Heterogeneous signal
    - Focal hyperintensities (compared to fat)
    - Curvilinear areas of signal void
- STIR: Hyperintense (corresponds to lytic lesions on NECT)
- Contrast-enhanced T1WI
  - o Common: Mild/moderate diffuse enhancement
  - o Uncommon: Peripheral (rim) enhancement

Other Modality Findings
- Radiography
  - o Can be normal early
  - o Lytic multicystic-appearing lesion +/- vertical dense striations
  - o Pathologic compression fracture common
- Radionuclide scans: Intense uptake (but can be normal early)

Imaging Recommendations
- Standard MR + STIR
- Scan entire spine!
- CT-guided biopsy/fine needle aspiration

Differential Diagnosis

Multiple Myeloma
- Second lesion found in 33% of cases with presumed spine SBP

Metastasis
- May be indistinguishable from SBP
- Posterior element involvement **not** useful in differentiating from SBP
- Doesn't involve disc or adjacent vertebrae

Benign (Osteoporotic) Compression Fracture
- Common in older patients, including those with SBP and MM
- 50-60% of compression fractures in MM appear benign on MR

- Signal intensity (subacute/chronic fxs) like normal marrow

Vertebral Hemangioma (VH)

- Aggressive VHs that mimic SBP, metastases are rare
- Marrow signal of aggressive VH may resemble SBP, metastases (most benign VHs are hyperintense on both T1-, T2WI)
- Intense enhancement

Pathology

General

- General Path Comments
  - o Marrow infiltrated with neoplastic plasma cells
- Genetics
  - o Unknown for SBP
  - o In situ hybridization studies show cytogenetic abnormalities in 80-90% of MM patients
    - Chromosome 13 deletion most common
    - Other: Chromosome 11q, miscellaneous translocations
    - Correlated with poor prognosis
- Etiology-Pathogenesis
  - o Malignant plasma cell disorder
  - o Monoclonal gammopathy
- Epidemiology
  - o Solitary bone plasmacytic lesions represent 3-5% of monoclonal gammopathies
  - o Spine is most common site

Gross Pathologic-Surgical Features

- Compressed vertebra with gray-purple fatty marrow replacement

Microscopic Features

- Monotonous collection of neoplastic plasma cells
  - o Eccentric, round, pleomorphic nuclei with "clock-face" chromatin
  - o Rich basophilic cytoplasm

Staging or Grading Criteria

- SBPs considered clinical stage I Durie/Salmon lesions
- Imaging shows normal bone or only SBP

Clinical Issues

Presentation

- Can be asymptomatic
- Most common symptom = pain
- Epidural extension, pathologic fracture may cause cord compression

Natural History

- SBPs typically have indolent course (median survival = 10y)

Treatment

- XRT
- Some asymptomatic patients with stage I MM not treated until more aggressive disease demonstrated at clinical follow-up

Prognosis

- SBPs are very radiosensitive (chance of cure if early dx, XRT)

Selected References
1.   Avva R et al: CT-guided biopsy of focal lesions in patients with multiple myeloma may reveal new and more aggressive cytogenetic abnormalities. AJNR 22: 781-5, 2001
2.   Shah BK et al: Magnetic resonance imaging of spinal plasmacytoma. Clin Radiol 55: 439-45, 2000
3.   Lecouvet F et al: Vertebral compression fractures in multiple myeloma. Radiol 204: 195-9, 1997

Lymphoma

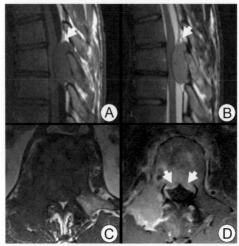

Sagittal T1- and T2WIs (A, B) show lymphoma with "cap" of epidural fat (arrows). Axial pre- (C), post-contrast T1WIs (D) in another case show marrow replacement, enhancing tumor extending into epidural space ("draped curtain" sign, arrows).

Key Facts
- Multiple types, variable imaging manifestations
  - Spinal epidural lymphoma (SEL)
  - Osseous lymphoma
  - Lymphomatous meningitis (LM)
  - Intramedullary lymphoma
- Secondary > primary involvement
  - 30% of systemic lymphomas have skeletal involvement
  - Primary osseous lymphoma = 3-4% of all malignant bone tumors
- Extradural > intradural > intramedullary

Imaging Findings
<u>General Features</u>
- Best imaging clue(s)
  - SEL: Enhancing epidural mass +/- vertebral involvement
  - Osseous lymphoma: Ivory vertebra (but rare!)
  - Lymphomatous meningitis (LM): Smooth/nodular pial enhancement
  - Intramedullary lymphoma: Poorly-defined enhancing mass
<u>CT Findings (SEL)</u>
- NECT: Epidural homogeneous, slightly dense mass, +/- bone involvement
- CECT: Homogeneous enhancement
<u>CT Findings (Osseous)</u>
- NECT: Lytic, permeative bone destruction; may cross disc spaces; +/- soft tissue mass; often spreads over multiple levels
<u>MR Findings (SEL)</u>
- T1WI: Isointense homogeneous epidural mass (often multisegmental +/- extends through foramina)
- T2WI: Iso/hyperintense (to cord)
- Contrast enhanced T1WI: Enhances intensely, uniformly

Lymphoma

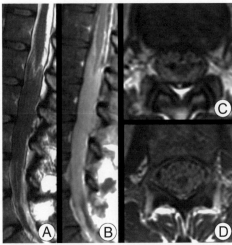

Sagittal T2- and post-contrast T1WI (A, B), axial post-contrast T1WI (C, D) show diffuse thickening and enhancement of cauda equina ("lymphomatous meningitis").

MR Findings (Osseous)
- T1WI: Hypointense to normal marrow (+/- epidural extension)
- T2WI: Variable; iso/hyperintense
- Contrast enhanced T1WI: Diffuse uniform enhancement

MR Findings (Lymphomatous Meningitis)
- T1/T2WI: Thick nerve roots +/- focal nodules (isointense with cord)
- Contrast enhanced T1WI: Roots enhance

MR Findings (Intramedullary)
- T1WI: Mass usually isointense to spinal cord
- T2WI: Hyperintense with surrounding edema
- Contrast-enhanced T1WI: Variable: patchy/confluent, infiltrating/discrete

Other Modality Findings
- Radiography
  - Bone destruction (30-40%)
  - Rare: "Ivory" vertebral body, vertebra plana

Imaging Recommendations
- MRI with contrast-enhanced, fat-saturated T1WI (STIR helpful)

Differential Diagnosis
Epidural Disease That May Mimic SEL
- Hematoma (heterogeneous > homogeneous signal)
- Abscess (rim > solid enhancement, central low signal common)
- Metastasis (epidural met without bone involvement rare)

Osseous Lymphoma Mimics
- Metastasis (destructive, +/- soft-tissue mass)
- E.G. (vertebra plana; younger patients)

Lymphomatous Meningitis Mimics
- Other neoplastic/granulomatous or infectious meningitides

Intramedullary Lymphoma Mimics
- Ependymoma (hemorrhage, cysts common)
- Astrocytoma (multisegmental; cysts common)

- Metastasis (usually round, more sharply delineated)

Pathology
General
- General Path Comments
  o SEL: Thoracic > lumbar > cervical
  o Common: Epidural extension from adjacent vertebral/paraspinous disease
  o Osseous lymphoma: Long bones > spine
  o Intramedullary lymphoma
    ▪ Cervical > thoracic > lumbar
    ▪ Can be primary or from systemic disease
- Etiology-Pathogenesis
  o CNS lymphoma may be primary or secondary (hematogenous or direct geographic extension)
  o AIDS/transplant patients predisposed to CNS lymphoma
  o EBV plays role in immunocompromised
- Epidemiology
  o NHL >> Hodgkin's disease (HD); 80-90% are B cell
  o Primary SEL= 1-7% of NHL; 10-30% of epidural malignancies
  o Secondary SEL in 5% of patients with systemic lymphoma
  o Primary osseous lymphoma = 3-4% of malignant bone tumors
  o Bone marrow involvement in 25-50% NHL patients, 5-15% HD
  o Epidural/vertebral involvement related to hematogenous metastatic involvement or local spread from adjacent lymph nodes
  o Intramedullary lymphoma = 3% of CNS lymphoma
  o LM nearly always occurs as spread from intracranial lymphoma

Gross Pathologic-Surgical Features
- Varies from discrete mass to poorly-marginated infiltrative disease

Microscopic Features
- Neoplastic lymphocytes in marrow, meninges; pack perivascular spaces

Staging or Grading Criteria
- CNS lymphoma >85% NHL (B-cell >>> T-cell), Hodgkin's disease rare

Clinical Issues
Presentation
- Adults (peak = 4th-7th decade), slight male predominance
- Most common presenting symptom = back pain
- SEL may cause cord compression
- Intramedullary = myelopathy (weakness, numbness, etc)

Natural History
- Cord compression occurs in up to 5-10% of systemic lymphomas
- Markedly sensitive to chemotherapy/XRT

Treatment
- XRT +/- chemotherapy (intrathecal for LM), +/- surgery

Prognosis
- Generally poor in CNS; primary osseous lymphoma best

Selected References
1. Koeller KK et al: Neoplasms of the spinal cord and filum terminale: Radiologic–Pathologic correlation. RadioGraphics 20:1721-49, 2000
2. Mulligan ME et al: Imaging features of primary lymphoma of bone. AJR 173:1691-7, 1999
3. Boukobza M et al: Primary vertebral and spinal epidural non-Hodgkin's lymphoma with spinal cord compression. Neuroradiology 38:333-7, 1996

Extradural Metastases

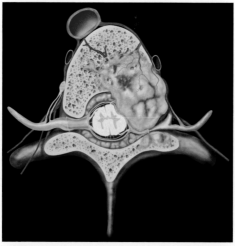

Axial graphic depicts extradural metastasis. Permeative, destructive mass erodes pedicle and posterior vertebral body, extends into epidural space, compresses cord.

Key Facts
- Spine metastases found in 5-10% of cancer patients
- High intensity lesion (STIR) in posterior vertebra/pedicle
- May cause pathologic fracture, cord compression

Imaging Findings
General Features
- Best imaging clue: Lesion destroys posterior cortex, pedicle

CT Findings
- NECT
  - Lytic, permeative destructive lesion(s)
    - Posterior vertebral body involved in almost all cases
    - 80% anterior body
    - 60% pedicle
    - 20% spinous, transverse processes and/or laminae
  - Location proportionate to red marrow (L>T>C spine)
  - +/- paraspinous/epidural soft tissue mass
  - Uncommon patterns
    - Diffuse sclerosis ("ivory" vertebra)
    - Lytic lesion with sclerotic rim
- CECT: Enhancement often not detectable

MR Findings
- Signal intensity **different** from uninvolved marrow
- T1WI
  - Hypointense
    - Solitary or multiple focal lesions
    - Diffuse involvement/replacement of fatty marrow causes generalized vertebral low signal (discs are "brighter" than bone)
  - Cortex (especially posterior), pedicle destroyed
  - Intervertebral discs generally spared

Extradural Metastases

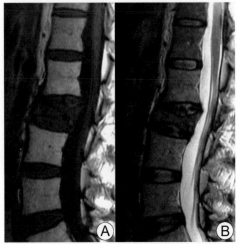

Sagittal T1- (A) and T2WI (B) in a patient with breast cancer and back pain show diffuse marrow infiltration, compression fracture of L2. Presumed metastasis.

- o May cause pathologic fracture with paraspinal/epidural mass
  - ▪ Usually involves more than one quadrant
  - ▪ "Draped curtain" sign = tumor spreads posteriorly into epidural space with relative midline sparing (at PLL)(see **Lymphoma** dx)
- T2WI: Hypo/isointense to normal marrow
- Short tau inversion recovery (STIR): Hyperintense
- DWI: Hyperintense (efficacy controversial)

Other Modality Findings
- Radiography (requires 50%-70% bone destruction for detection)
  - o AP: Absent ("missing") pedicle, +/- paraspinous soft tissue mass
  - o Lateral: Destroyed posterior cortical line
- Scintigraphy
  - o Tc^{99m} SPECT has high sensitivity
- Myelography, myelo-CT (use only if MR unavailable)
  - o Extradural compression
  - o "Block" (ill-defined "feathered" edge to contrast column)
- Biochemical markers indicate presence/extent of skeletal metastases

Imaging Recommendations
- Scan entire spine!
  - o Standard MRI + STIR or fat-suppressed T2WI (scan entire spine)
  - o Contrast-enhanced, fat-saturated T1WI
  - o Water-suppressed T1WI if contrast not available
- Radionuclide studies if equivocal

Differential Diagnosis

Hematopoietic Malignancy
- Plasmacytoma, multiple myeloma (MM), lymphoma, leukemia
- Radionuclide studies negative/equivocal in 25% of MM
- Diffuse marrow involvement more common than metastasis

Benign (Osteoporotic) vs. Malignant Compression Fracture
- May be difficult to distinguish acute osteoporotic fx (DWI may be helpful)

- o 1/3 of fxs in patients with known primary tumor are benign
- o 1/4 of fxs in apparently osteopenic patients are from malignant disease
- Marrow signal with late subacute/chronic benign fractures similar to normal marrow (suppresses on STIR)

Inhomogeneous Marrow
- Focal/irregular, patchy fatty marrow in older patients
- Intact pedicle, posterior vertebral cortex

Avascular Necrosis
- Vacuum cleft below endplate, usually anterior vertebral body

Pathology
General
- General Path Comments
  - o Marrow initially infiltrated, trabeculae destroyed, then cortex
- Etiology-Pathogenesis
  - o Hematogenous dissemination (arterial or venous via Batson's plexus) > perineural, lymphatic, CSF spread
  - o Marrow infiltration precedes osseous destruction
    - ▪ Posterior vertebral body first, then pedicle
  - o Primary tumor (adults)
    - ▪ Lung, breast, prostate, kidney most common spinal metastases
    - ▪ Unknown primary in 15%-25%
  - o Primary tumor (children): Sarcomas (Ewing, neuroblastoma), hematologic malignancies
- Epidemiology
  - o Vertebral metastases
    - ▪ 10-40% of patients with systemic cancer
    - ▪ Account for 40% of all bone metastases
  - o Epidural spinal cord compression (ESCC) in 5% of adults with systemic cancers (70% solitary, 30% multiple sites)
  - o ESCC occurs in 5% of children with malignant solid tumors
    - ▪ Invade canal via neural foramen
    - ▪ Circumferential cord compression common

Gross Pathologic-Surgical Features
- Softened, eroded bone +/- adjacent soft tissue mass

Microscopic Features
- Varies with histology of primary, osteoclastic/blastic response

Clinical Issues
Presentation
- Progressive axial, referred, or radicular pain
- ESCC may cause paralysis, sensory loss, incontinence

Natural History
- Relentless, progressive; pathologic fracture, ESCC may ensue

Treatment
- XRT, surgical decompression (options = vertebroplasty, embolization)

Prognosis
- Varies with histology of primary lesion

Selected References
1. Castillo M et al: Diffusion-weighted MR imaging offers no advantage over routine noncontrast MR imaging in the detection of vertebral metastases. AJNR 21: 948-53, 2000
2. Chamberlain MC et al: Epidural spinal cord compression. Neuro-oncol 1: 120-3, 1999
3. Vanel D et al: MRI of bone metastases. Eur Radiol 8: 1345-51, 1998

Spinal Meningioma

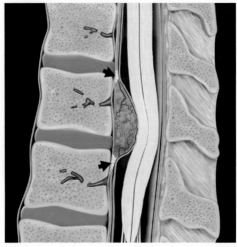

Sagittal graphic depicts spinal meningioma. The intradural/extramedullary location is typical. The tumor has a broad dural base, mild reactive dural thickening (arrows), and moderate cord compression. The meningioma is covered by a thin layer of arachnoid and has a sharply-defined border ("meniscus") defined by CSF.

Key Facts
- Definition: Slow growing, benign, dural-based tumor
- Second most common intradural extramedullary neoplasm
- Most common site = thoracic (80%)
- Imaging: Intradural, extramedullary enhancing mass +/- dural "tail"

Imaging Findings
General Features
- Best imaging clue: Enhancing intradural/extramedullary mass + dural tail
  - 90% intradural (10% extradural and/or "dumbbell")
  - Ca++< 5%

CT Findings
- NECT: Iso- to hyperdense mass (compared to muscle)
- CECT: Strong homogeneous enhancement

MR Findings
- T1WI: Isointense (to spinal cord)
- T2WI
  - Iso/hyperintense
  - May be hypointense if densely calcified
  - Very vascular meningioma may have prominent "flow voids"
- Contrast-enhanced T1WI
  - Intense, homogeneous enhancement
  - +/- broad-based dural attachment ("tail" less common than intracranial)

Other Modality Findings
- Myelography, CT myelography
  - Sharp meniscus of contrast caps lesion (classic for intradural, extramedullary mass)
  - Ipsilateral subarachnoid space widened (cord, roots displaced away from mass)

Spinal Meningioma

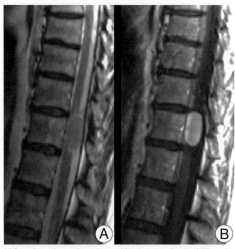

A 56-year-old female with myelopathy and back pain. Sagittal T2 and post-contrast T1WIs (A, B) show an intradural, extramedullary thoracic mass. Note the intense homogeneous enhancement characteristic for meningioma. A "dural tail" is not seen in this case.

Imaging Recommendations
- Contrast enhanced MRI
- CT (if densely calcified)

Differential Diagnosis

Schwannoma
- Very hyperintense on T2WI
- Cystic change, hemorrhage more common
- No dural attachment

Other Intradural Extramedullary Masses
- Paraganglioma (rare)
- Epidermoid (signal usually = CSF)
- Arachnoid cyst (like CSF, doesn't enhance)
- Intradural metastasis (often multiple)

Lymphoma
- Solitary intradural mass uncommon

Pathology

General
- General Path Comments
  - o Intracranial: Spine meningiomas = 8:1
  - o Thoracic (80%)>> cervical (16%) > lumbar (4%)
- Genetics (almost all have chromosome 22 abnormalities)
  - o Most are solitary, sporadic
  - o Multiple meningiomas
    - ▪ NF-2
    - ▪ Multiple meningiomatosis
    - ▪ Familial clear cell meningioma syndrome

Spinal Meningioma

- Etiology-Pathogenesis
  - o Arise from arachnoid cap cell rests
- Epidemiology
  - o Second most common intradural extramedullary tumor
    - 25% of primary spinal tumors
  - o F:M = 4:1

Gross Pathologic-Surgical Features
- Firm, well demarcated, lobulated/rounded mass with dural attachment
- Expands centripetally within dural sac

Microscopic Features
- Most are "typical" meningiomas
  - o Common histologic subtypes
    - Most common = psammomatous type with Ca++ concretions
    - Meningothelial
    - Fibrous
    - Transitional
  - o Less common = angiomatous, microcystic, rhabdoid, clear cell, chordoid, etc.
- Rare
  - o Atypical (increased mitoses, cellularity, etc.)
  - o Anaplastic (malignant)

Staging or Grading Criteria
- > 95% WHO grade I

Clinical Issues

Presentation
- Most common presenting symptom = pain
  - o Other = motor/sensory deficits, gait disturbance
- Peak incidence = fifth/sixth decades (younger if NF2)
- > 80% female

Natural History
- Slow growing, compresses but doesn't invade adjacent structures

Treatment
- Complete surgical resection
- +/- XRT (subtotal resection, aggressive tumors)

Prognosis
- Excellent prognosis with complete excision
- Recurrence rate up to 40% at 5 years in patients with incomplete resection, en plaque, and infiltrative meningioma

Selected References
1. Louis DN et al: Meningiomas. In Kleihues P, Cavanee WK (eds), Tumours of the Nervous System, 176-84, IARC Press, 2000
2. Klekamp J et al: Surgical results for spinal meningiomas. Surg Neurol 52: 552-62, 1999
3. Solero CL et al: Spinal meinigiomas: Review of 174 operated cases. Neurosurg 125: 153-60, 1989

Spinal Schwannoma

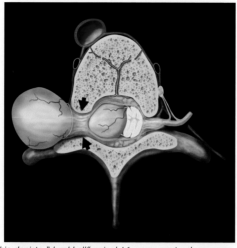

Axial graphic depicts "dumbbell" spinal L1 nerve root schwannoma. The well-delineated tumor has both intra- and extradural components. Note compression of the distal cord, enlargement of the neural foramen (arrows).

Key Facts

- Schwannoma = most common intradural extramedullary mass
- Extradural, "dumbbell" (combined intra-, extradural) tumors also occur
- Most common symptom = pain
- Clinical presentation can mimic HNP!

Imaging Findings

General Features

- Best imaging clue: Well-delineated, enhancing, spinal nerve root mass
  - o 70-75% intradural extramedullary
  - o 15% extradural
  - o 15% "dumbbell"
- Majority are small (a few mm up to 1-2 vertebral segments)
- Multisegmental giant schwannomas do occur
- Difficult to distinguish schwannoma, other nerve sheath tumors (e.g., neurofibroma) on basis of imaging findings alone

CT Findings

- NECT
  - o Sharply-delineated mass
  - o Isodense with cord, nerve roots
    - Cysts common
    - Gross hemorrhage uncommon
    - Ca++ rare
  - o Adjacent bone erosion, remodeling common
    - Enlarged neural foramen with "dumbbell" lesion
    - Large lesions may expand canal, cause posterior vertebral body scalloping
- CECT
  - o Moderate solid/rim enhancement

Spinal Schwannoma

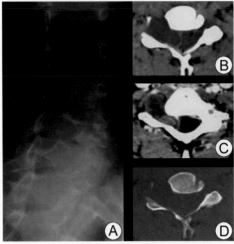

This patient presented with right arm pain. (A) Oblique cervical spine radiograph shows C6-7 neural foramen enlargement. Axial CT scans without (B) and with (C) contrast show a mixed cystic/solid partially enhancing "dumbbell" tumor. Bone window (D) demonstrates smooth foraminal enlargement. Schwannoma.

MR Findings
- T1WI
  - Most are hypointense relative to cord, roots
  - Pigmented (melanotic) schwannoma may have short T1
- T2WI
  - 75% hyperintense, 40% cysts, 10% hemorrhage
  - Occasional: "Target" pattern (high signal rim, low intensity center)
- Almost always enhance intensely
  - Can be uniform or heterogeneous pattern

Other Modality Findings
- DSA: Variable vascularity (none to moderate)

Imaging Recommendations
- Contrast-enhanced, fat-suppressed MR
- Scan entire spine in asymptomatic patients with suspected NF-2!

Differential Diagnosis

Schwannoma vs. Neurofibroma
- May be difficult to distinguish on imaging alone

Myxopapillary Ependymoma
- Usually larger, more vascular
- Hemorrhage more common
- May be indistinguishable from giant schwannoma

Conjoined Nerve Root/Sleeve
- CSF signal intensity
- Doesn't enhance
- Smaller than normal lateral recess/neural foramen below/above involved level

Extruded Disc Fragments
- May extend down root sleeve, mimic neoplasm

Spinal Schwannoma

- Usually hypo- (not hyperintense), doesn't enhance

Pathology
General
- General Path Comments
  - Mass spreads, deviates nerve fascicles
- Genetics
  - Sporadic: Inactivating mutations of NF2 gene in 60%
  - Inherited tumor syndromes
    - NF2: Multiple schwannomas; chromosome 22q mutations
    - Schwannomatosis: Multiple peripheral schwannomas in absence of other NF2 features
    - Carney complex: Mendelian-dominant (chromosome 17); melanotic schwannoma, cutaneous myxomas, potentially life-threatening cardiac myxomas, pigmented adrenal tumors
- Etiology-Pathogenesis
  - Inactivation of NF2 gene (encodes for merlin protein)
- Epidemiology
  - 30% of primary spine neoplasms
  - Usually solitary unless inherited tumor syndrome
  - M = F
  - Peak incidence = 4th-6th decades
  - Multiple asymptomatic spinal schwannomas occur in children with NF-2
Gross Pathologic-Surgical Features
- Circumscribed, well-encapsulated, light tan/yellow, round/ovoid mass
- May have cysts; gross hemorrhage, frank necrosis uncommon
Microscopic Features
- 3-layered capsule (fibrous layer, nerve tissue, transitional layer)
- Schwann cell = neoplastic element
- Classic "biphasic" pattern
  - Compact, elongated cells with occasional palisading (Antoni A)
  - Less cellular, loosely textured, often lipidized (Antoni B)
- May contain melanin (50% have Carney complex)
Staging or Grading Criteria
- WHO grade I

Clinical Issues
Presentation
- Pain (can mimic sciatica, disc herniation)
Natural History
- Slowly growing
- Malignant degeneration rarely occurs (risk higher with NF-2)
Treatment
- Total microsurgical resection
Prognosis
- No recurrence (NF2, schwannomatosis may develop new lesions)

Selected References
1. Hasegawa M et al: Surgical pathology of spinal schwannomas. Neurosurg 6: 1388-93, 2001
2. Woodruff JM et al: Schwannoma. In Kleihues P, Cavenee WK (eds). Tumours of the Nervous System, 164-6. IARC Press, 2000
3. Murphey MD et al: Imaging of musculoskeletal neurogenic tumors: Radiologic-pathologic correlation. RadioGraphics 19: 1253-80, 1999

Spinal Neurofibroma

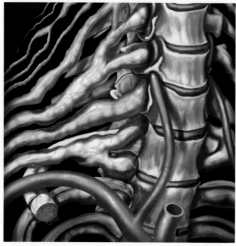

Graphic depiction of plexiform neurofibromas in NF-1. Bulky multilevel tumors involve the cervical nerve roots and brachial plexus. The neural foramina are enlarged.

Key Facts
- 90% of neurofibromas (NF) occur as sporadic, solitary tumors
- NFs can be localized, diffuse or plexiform
- Multiple plexiform NFs occur as part of NF-1, an inherited tumor syndrome
- 50% of malignant peripheral nerve sheath tumors (MPNSTs) are associated with NF-1

Imaging Findings
General Features
- Best imaging clue: Bulky multilevel spinal nerve root tumors in patient with cutaneous stigmata of NF-1
CT Findings
- NECT
  - Hypodense focal/fusiform enlargement of nerve root(s)
  - +/- enlarged neural foramina
- CECT: Mild/moderate enhancement
MR Findings
- T1WI: Usually isointense with spinal cord, nerve roots
- T2WI
  - Iso/hyperintense
  - "Target sign"
    - Hyperintense rim, low/intermediate center
    - Suggests neurogenic tumor but is not pathognomonic for NF
- Variable enhancement (usually mild/moderate, relatively uniform)
Other Modality Findings
- Radionuclide studies: MPNSTs may show intense uptake
Imaging Recommendations
- MR (include fat-saturated T2WI or STIR sequence, contrast)

Spinal Neurofibroma

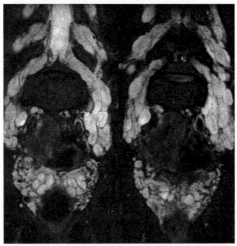

Coronal STIR images in a patient with NF-1 show multilevel plexiform neurofibromas involving the spinal and pelvic nerves.

Differential Diagnosis

Schwannoma
- May be indistinguishable from solitary NF on imaging studies
- "Target" sign more common with NF than schwannoma

Meningocele
- Cystic, follows CSF density/signal intensity
- Fills with intrathecal contrast

Congenital Hypertrophic Polyradiculoneuropathies
- Charcot-Marie-Tooth, Dejerine-Sottas disease
- Can mimic plexiform NF on imaging studies
- No cutaneous stigmata of NF-1

Chronic Interstitial Demyelinating Polyneuropathy (CIDP)
- Caused by repeated episodes of demyelination, remyelination
- "Onion" skin layered enlargement of spinal, peripheral nerves
- Can mimic plexiform NF on imaging studies
- No cutaneous stigmata of NF-1

Miscellaneous Causes of Multiple, Enlarged, Enhancing Spinal Nerves
- Inflammatory neuritis
  - CMV radiculopathy in HIV+
  - Mechanical/chemical nerve root irritation (HNP, postoperative)
- Neoplastic neuritis
  - Lymphoma
  - Leptomeningeal metastases

Pathology

General
- General Path Comments
  - Variable appearance from circumscribed nodular masses to diffusely infiltrating tumors
- Genetics

Spinal Neurofibroma

- o Germline mutations of NF1 gene
  - ▪ Loss of remaining wild-type NF1 allele in patients with NF-1
  - ▪ NF1 genetic alterations probable with sporadic NFs
- • Epidemiology
  - o 5% of all benign soft tissue tumors
  - o Peak presentation at 20-30y
  - o No gender predilection

Gross Pathologic-Surgical Features
- • Three gross types of NFs recognized
  - o Localized
    - ▪ 90% of NFs
    - ▪ Solitary fusiform mass, usually < 5 cm
    - ▪ Not associated with NF-1
  - o Diffuse
    - ▪ Infiltrating tumor of children, young adults
    - ▪ Usually affects subcutaneous tissues of head, neck
    - ▪ Rarely involves spinal nerves
    - ▪ 90% sporadic, isolated, not associated with NF-1
  - o Plexiform
    - ▪ Pathognomonic for NF-1
    - ▪ Usually bilateral, multilevel
    - ▪ Often affects sciatic nerve, brachial plexus
    - ▪ Long, bulky, ropy expansion of affected nerves ("bag of worms")

Microscopic Features
- • Neoplastic Schwann cells + fibroblasts
- • Collagen fibers, mucoid/myxoid matrix
- • Tumor, nerve fascicles intermixed
- • S-100 positive
- • Mitotic figures rare in NFs

Staging or Grading Criteria
- • NFs are WHO grade I
- • MPNSTs are WHO grade III/IV

Clinical Issues

Presentation
- • Mass (focal or diffusely infiltrating) common, pain rare
- • +/- stigmata of NF-1 (café-au-lait spots, axillary freckling)

Natural History
- • Slow-growing
- • Malignant transformation to MPNSTs
  - o Rare with sporadic NFs
  - o 5% of plexiform NFs

Treatment
- • Resection of sporadic/solitary NF; plexiform NFs usually nonsurgical

Prognosis
- • Both plexiform, solitary NFs of major nerves can be precursors to MPNSTs

Selected References
1. Simoens WA et al: MR features of peripheral nerve sheath tumors: can a calculated index compete with radiologist's experience? Eur Radiol 11: 250-7, 2001
2. Woodruff JM et al: Neurofibroma. In: Kleihues P, Cavenee WK (eds), Tumors of the Nervous System, 167-8, IARC Press, 2000
3. Murphey MD et al: Imaging of musculoskeletal neurogenic tumors: Radiologic-pathologic correlation. RadioGraphics 19: 1253-80, 1999

Myxopapillary Ependymoma

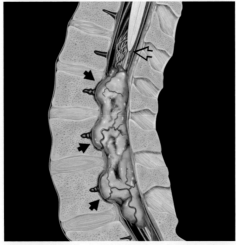

Sagittal graphic of cauda equina myxopapillary ependymoma. The vascular mass extends over three segments and expands the canal, causing posterior vertebral body scalloping (small arrows). Note evidence for old intratumoral hemorrhage as well as acute nonaneurysmal SAH (open arrow).

Key Facts
- Distinct type of slow-growing ependymoma
- Most common tumor of conus/cauda equina/filum terminale
- Cysts, hemorrhage common (may cause acute nonaneurysmal SAH)
- Often presents with back pain
  - Can be missed if scans don't include conus!

Imaging Findings
General Features
- Best imaging clue: Enhancing cauda equina mass with hemorrhage
CT Findings
- NECT
  - Isodense intradural mass
  - +/- bony canal focal expansion
    - Thinned pedicles
    - Widened interpediculate distance
    - Scalloped vertebral bodies
    - May enlarge, extend through, neural foramina
- CECT: Enhances strongly, uniformly
MR Findings
- T1WI: Usually isointense with cord
- T2WI: Almost always hyperintense to cord
- Enhances strongly
- Hemorrhagic residua common
  - 70% of intradural spine tumors with blood are ependymomas!
  - May cause acute nonaneurysmal SAH, superficial siderosis (low signal rim on surface of cerebellum, brainstem, cord)
- Cysts, vascular "flow voids" common
- Rare: May occur as destructive extradural sacrococcygeal lesion

Myxopapillary Ependymoma

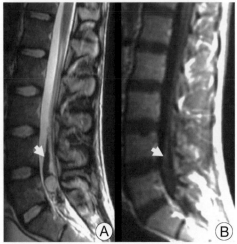

A 12-year-old male presented with back pain, acute subarachnoid hemorrhage. Three cerebral angiograms were negative for aneurysm. Sagittal T2WI (A) and post-contrast T1WI (B) demonstrate an enhancing cauda equina mass with subacute hemorrhage (arrows). Myxopapillary ependymoma was found at surgery.

Other Modality Findings
- CT with intrathecal contrast/myelography
  - Well-delineated lobulated/ovoid mass below conus/along filum
  - "Meniscus" of contrast delineates intradural extramedullary mass

Imaging Recommendations
- **Always scan the conus in patients with back pain!!**
- Scan up to at least mid-thoracic spine if conus lesion found

Differential Diagnosis

Nerve Sheath Tumor (NST)
- Large, multilevel NST may be indistinguishable
- Usually extends through neural foramina
- Hemorrhage occurs but less common

Meningioma
- Usually isointense with cord on T1-, T2WI
- More common in thoracic, cervical spine (conus/filum location unusual)
- Usually doesn't hemorrhage, expand canal, erode bone

Paraganglioma
- Rare tumor of cauda equina
- May be highly vascular, indistinguishable from myxopapillary ependymoma
- Usually smaller

Other Tumors
- Hemangioblastoma (usually intramedullary)
- Subependymoma (uncommon)

Pathology

General
- General Path Comments

Myxopapillary Ependymoma

- o Occurs almost exclusively in conus/cauda equina/filum terminale
- o Slow-growing, often encapsulated
- o Usually spans 2-4 vertebral segments
  - May become huge, fill entire lumbosacral sac
- o 10-40% have multiple lesions
- Genetics: No consistent alterations reported
- Etiology-Pathogenesis
  - o Originates from ependymal glia of filum
- Epidemiology
  - o 10-15% of all ependymomas
  - o 80-90% of filum terminale tumors
  - o M: F = 2:1
  - o Broad age range
    - Reported at all ages
    - Peak 3rd-4th decades

Gross Pathologic-Surgical Features
- Soft, lobulated, grayish tumor
- Noninfiltrating, often encapsulated
- May be highly vascular

Microscopic Features
- Elongated/cuboidal tumor cells with radial perivascular arrangement
- Fibrous/mucoid matrix
- Cysts, hemorrhage common
- Absent/low mitotic activity (MIB 0.4-1.6%)
- GFAP, S-100, vimentin positive
- Cytokeratins negative

Staging or Grading Criteria
- WHO grade I
- May have local seeding, subarachnoid dissemination
- No malignant degeneration

Clinical Issues

Presentation
- Most common symptom = back pain
  - o May mimic HNP!
  - o Average duration of symptoms prior to diagnosis = 2y
- Leg weakness, bowel dysfunction in 20%-25%

Natural History
- Late recurrence/distant metastases uncommon after complete resection
- Risk of local recurrence if resection incomplete

Treatment
- Resection
- +/- XRT, adjuvant therapy for multifocal lesions

Prognosis
- Excellent with complete resection

Selected References
1. Wiestler OD et al: Myxopapillary ependymoma. In Kleihues P, Cavenee WK (eds): Tumors of the Central Nervous System, 78-9. IARC Press, 2000
2. Friedman DP et al: Neuroradiology case of the day. RadioGraphics 18: 794-8, 1998
3. Wippold FJ II et al: MR imaging of myxopapillary ependymoma. AJR 165: 1263-7, 1995

Spinal Paraganglioma

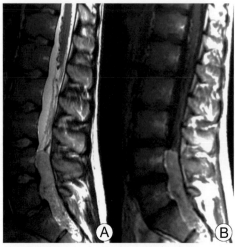

A 22-year-old male with low back pain was imaged to "rule out disc herniation."
Sagittal T2- (A) and post-contrast T1WI (B) disclosed a very vascular enhancing
mass of the cauda equina. Note prominent "flow voids." Preoperative diagnosis was
myxopapillary ependymoma. Paraganglioma was found at surgery.

Key Facts
- Synonyms
  - Chemodectoma, glomus tumor (terminology based on anatomic site)
- Spine = rare extra-adrenal site of paraganglioma (PG)
- Almost always in cauda equina
- Endocrinologically silent (causes back/extremity pain)
- Imaging features nonspecific (vascular intradural extramedullary mass)

Imaging Findings
General Features
- Best imaging clue: Vascular cauda equina mass
- May be indistinguishable from other intradural extramedullary tumors
CT Findings
- NECT
  - Usually normal
  - Large tumors may show bony remodeling, even erosion
  - Rare presentation = destructive intraosseous mass (usually in sacrum)
- CECT: May demonstrate enhancing mass below conus/along filum
MR Findings
- T1WI
  - Well-delineated round/ovoid/lobulated mass
  - Iso-, mixed iso/hypointense compared to cord
  - Prominent "flow voids" common
- T2WI: Hyperintense +/- blood products, hemosiderin rim or "cap"
- Contrast-enhanced T1WI: Intense homogeneous enhancement
  - Rare: Demonstrates multiple "uphill" intradural metastases
Other Modality Findings
- Myelography, CT myelography
  - Smooth/lobulated intradural extramedullary mass
  - +/- serpentine filling defects (large arteries, draining veins)

Spinal Paraganglioma

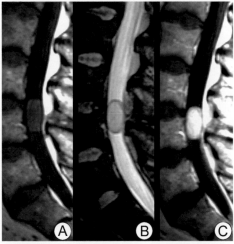

Sagittal pre-contrast T1- (A) and T2WI (B) in a patient with back pain show a well-delineated cauda equina mass that enhances intensely after contrast administration (C). Preoperative diagnosis was schwannoma vs. ependymoma. Paraganglioma was found at surgery (case courtesy L. Hutchings).

<u>Imaging Recommendations</u>
- Contrast-enhanced MRI (do entire spine!)

Differential Diagnosis
<u>Myxopapillary Ependymoma</u>
- May be indistinguishable on imaging studies, standard light microscopy
- Immunohistochemistry distinguishes PG from ependymoma, other tumors
<u>Schwannoma</u>
- Usually less vascular, hemorrhage less common than PG
- Vascular schwannoma may be indistinguishable
<u>Meningioma</u>
- Thoracic > lumbar (even less common in cauda equina)
- Dural-based mass +/- reactive thickening ("tail" sign)
<u>Metastasis</u>
- Vascular intradural extramedullary metastasis may be indistinguishable

Pathology
<u>General</u>
- General Path Comments
  - Can be difficult to distinguish PG from ependymoma using only light microscopy, standard H & E stains
- Genetics
  - Sporadic: Cyto-, molecular genetics unknown
  - Familial
    - No reports of familial cauda equina PGs
    - Other extra-adrenal PGs can occur with MEN types 2A/2B, VHL
- Etiology-Pathogenesis
  - PGs originate from neural crest cells associated with segmental or collateral autonomic ganglia ("paraganglia") throughout body

Spinal Paraganglioma

- o "APUD" cell tumors (**A**mine **P**recursor **U**ptake and **D**ecarboxylation)
- o Histogenesis of spinal PGs debatable
  - Paraganglionic tissue not normally found in cauda equina
  - Peripheral neuroblasts in filum may undergo paraganglionic differentiation
- Epidemiology
  - o Most neural crest tumors occur in adrenal medulla (pheochromocytoma)
  - o 80%-90% of extra-adrenal paragangliomas occur in/near carotid body, jugular bulb
  - o Spine is uncommon site
  - o Cauda equina PGs may represent distinct subtype of extra-adrenal PG

Gross Pathologic-Surgical Features
- Encapsulated, soft, dark red-brown tumor
- Richly vascular

Microscopic Features
- Well-differentiated tumor (resembles normal paraganglia)
  - o Chief (type I) cells arranged in compact nests ("zellballen")
  - o Surrounded by inconspicuous single layer of sustentacular (type II) cells
- Round/oval nuclei with finely stippled chromatin, indistinct nucleoli
- Sinusoidal blood vessels (occasionally thick-walled, hyalinized)
- Immunohistochemistry + for synaptophysin
- E.M. shows dense core neurosecretory granules

Staging or Grading Criteria
- WHO grade I
- Rare aggressive, malignant spinal paragangliomas have been reported

Clinical Issues

Presentation
- Age at presentation
  - o Range from 13 to 70y
  - o Average = 45-50y
- Spinal paragangliomas have little/no secretory activity
- Most common symptom = back/lower extremity pain
- Other: Sensory/motor loss, bowel/bladder dysfunction
- Symptom duration varies from days to years

Natural History
- Slow-growing, generally benign behavior

Treatment
- Surgical excision usually curative

Prognosis
- Varies with tumor location (generally excellent for spinal PGs)
- Recurrence <5% after gross total removal

Selected References
1. Soffer D et al: Paraganglioma. In P Kleihues, WK Cavenee (eds), Tumours of the Nervous System, 112-4, IARC Press, 2000
2. Sundgren P et al: Paragangliomas of the spinal canal. Neuroradiol 41: 788-94, 1999
3. Rees JH et al: Paragangliomas of the cauda equina. IJNR 2: 242-50, 1996

Intradural Metastases

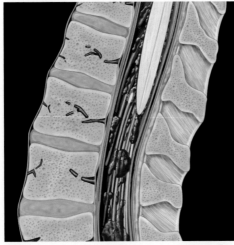

Intradural metastases involving the conus and cauda equina are illustrated. Note "sugarlike" coating of the cord and roots ("carcinomatous meningitis"). Small and occasionally large tumor nodules can be seen. In some cases, a solitary "drop metastasis" is present at the distal thecal sac.

Key Facts

- In adults, intradural << extradural spinal metastases
  - Leptomeningeal >> cord metastases
- In children, intradural > extradural metastases
- Classic imaging appearance = "carcinomatous meningitis"
- Can be caused by spread from intracranial neoplasm ("drop mets") or nonCNS primary tumor

Imaging Findings

General Features
- Best imaging clue: Smooth/nodular enhancement along cord, roots
- 4 basic patterns
  - Diffuse, thin, sheetlike coating of cord/roots ("carcinomatous meningitis")
  - Multifocal discrete nodules along cord/roots
  - "Rope-like" thickening of cauda equina
  - Solitary focal mass
    - At bottom of thecal sac
    - Intramedullary nodule

CT Findings
- NECT
  - Often normal; +/- bony/extradural tumor present
- CECT
  - Often normal

MR Findings
- T1WI
  - Metastases usually isointense with cord, roots
  - Extensive disease may fill thecal sac (see Lymphoma illustration)
    - CSF in sac has "ground glass" appearance
    - Nerve roots appear blurred, "smudged"

Intradural Metastases

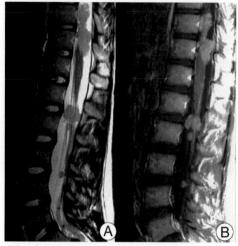

Sagittal T2- (A) and post-contrast T1WIs (B) in a patient with a pineal germinoma show multiple metastases coating the conus and cauda equina. Several large tumor nodules are present. Both "drop" metastases from CNS tumors as well as spread from extracranial primary neoplasms can cause this pattern.

- T2WI
  - Metastases usually isointense with cord, roots (hypointense to CSF)
- Contrast-enhanced T1WI
  - Strong enhancement
  - Pattern varies
    - "Sugar coating" of cord, roots
    - Single/multiple enhancing nodular masses
    - Round/ovoid intramedullary mass, often with ring-like pattern

Other Modality Findings
- Myelography, CT myelography
  - "Filling defects"
    - Single or multifocal nodules
    - Expanded cord, thickened nerve roots

Imaging Recommendations
- Image entire neuraxis!
  - High resolution T2WI
  - Contrast-enhanced, fat-suppressed T1WI
  - STIR (look for bony metastases)
- Do it **prior** to craniotomy!

Differential Diagnosis (Varies with Pattern)
Postoperative Change
- Subarachnoid blood, adhesions can mimic leptomeningeal mets
"Carcinomatous Meningitis"
- Pyogenic meningitis (clinical/laboratory findings helpful)
- Sarcoidosis
"Drop Metastases"
- Usually pathognomonic
- Multifocal primary tumor

- o Myxopapillary ependymoma
- o Hemangioblastoma
- o Astrocytoma (uncommon)

Thick Nerve Roots/Cauda Equina
- Congenital hypertrophic polyradiculoneuropathies
  - o Charcot-Marie-Tooth
  - o Dejerine-Sottas
- Chronic interstitial demyelinating polyneuropathy (CIDP)
- Chemotherapy-associated polyneuropathy
- AIDS-associated polyneuropathy (e.g., CMV)

Intramedullary Metastasis (Rare)
- Radiation-induced myelitis
- Primary cord tumor (met = focal nodule + edema > infiltrating mass)

Pathology

General
- General Path Comments
  - o Broad spectrum of primary neoplasms
- Etiology-Pathogenesis
  - o Hematogenous dissemination from extracranial neoplasm
    - Most are adenocarcinomas (lung, breast)
    - Other = non-Hodgkin lymphoma, leukemia
  - o "Drop" metastases from CNS primary tumor
    - Adults = anaplastic astrocytoma, GBM (0.5%-1% of cases)
    - Children = PNETs (medulloblastoma), ependymoma, choroid plexus tumors (both papillomas, carcinomas), germinomas
- Epidemiology
  - o 5% of all spinal metastases
  - o Prevalence increasing

Gross Pathologic-Surgical Features
- Varies with pattern, type of metastasis

Microscopic Features
- Varies with histology of primary neoplasm
- CSF usually positive in leptomeningeal metastatic disease; negative in intramedullary tumors

Clinical Issues

Presentation
- Varies; may be asymptomatic early
- Radiculopathy > myelopathy

Natural History
- Relentless progression typical

Treatment
- Radiation, chemotherapy

Prognosis
- Survival usually < 1y

Selected References
1. Markus JB: MRI of intramedullary spinal cord metastases. Clin Imaging 20: 238-42, 1996
2. Heinz R et al: Detection of CSF metastasis: CT myelography or MR? AJNR 16: 1147-51, 1995
3. Schuknecht B et al: Spinal leptomeningeal neoplastic disease. Eur Neurol 32: 11-6, 1992

Cord Astrocytoma

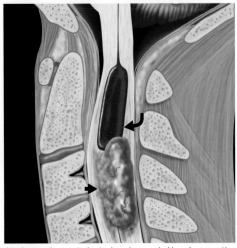

Sagittal graphic depicts the cervical spinal cord expanded by a large cystic astrocytoma. Note solid nodule (large arrow) with associated cyst (curved arrows). Growth pattern in cord astrocytomas is often eccentric and even occasionally exophytic. Multisegmental cord enlargement is typical.

Key Facts
- Second most common cord neoplasm
- Most common intramedullary tumor in children/young adults
- May cause painful scoliosis
- Usually low grade, grows slowly
- Infiltrative/eccentric, occasionally exophytic growth pattern

Imaging Findings
General Features
- Best imaging clue: Enhancing infiltrating cord mass in child
CT Findings
- NECT
  - Enlarged cord
  - +/- expansion, remodeling of bony canal
- CECT: Mild/moderate enhancement
MR Findings
- T1WI
  - Cord expansion
    - Usually < 4 segments
    - Occasionally multisegmental, even holocord (more common with pilocytic astrocytoma)
  - +/- cyst/syrinx (fluid slightly hyperintense to CSF)
  - Solid portion iso/mixed hypo/isointense
- T2WI
  - Hyperintense on PD, T2WI
- T1WI + contrast
  - Almost always enhances
    - Mild/moderate > intense enhancement
    - Partial > total enhancement
    - Inhomogeneous/infiltrating > homogeneous/sharply-delineated

Cord Astrocytoma

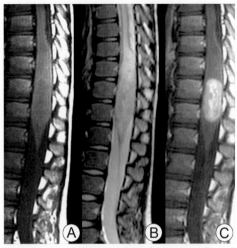

A 4-year-old male complained of leg pain. Sagittal pre-contrast T1- and T2WI (A, B) show multisegmental expansion of the distal thoracic spinal cord and conus. Contrast-enhanced T1WI (C) demonstrates an intensely enhancing, well-delineated tumor nodule. Mixed oligoastrocytoma was found at surgery.

Other Modality Findings
• Myelography: Expanded cord (nonspecific)
Imaging Recommendations
• Contrast-enhanced MR

Differential Diagnosis
Ependymoma
• Patients often older
• Intense, sharply delineated enhancement
• Central > eccentric growth pattern
• Hemorrhage common
Other Neoplasms
• Ganglioglioma, mixed glioma (may be indistinguishable)
• Hemangioblastoma, lymphoma, metastasis (older patients)
Syringohydromyelia
• Cyst fluid like CSF; no enhancement
Nonneoplastic Myelopathy
• Demyelinating disease (+/- patchy, ill-defined enhancement if acute)
• Cord ischemia/infarction (abrupt onset; risk factors include ASVD, HTN, diabetes, aortic dissection)

Pathology
General
• General Path Comments
  o Eccentric > central growth pattern
  o Bony canal often enlarged, remodeled
  o Cervical > thoracic
• Epidemiology

Cord Astrocytoma

- o Intramedullary spinal cord tumors (IMSCTs) = 5-10% of all CNS tumors
  - 20% of intraspinal neoplasms in adults
  - 30-35% of intraspinal neoplasms in children
- o 90-95% of IMSCTs are gliomas
  - Overall, ependymomas 2x astrocytoma
  - 60% of IMSCTs in children are astrocytomas, 30% ependymomas
  - Diffuse fibrillary > pilocytic astrocytoma
- o M: F = 1.3:1

Gross Pathologic-Surgical Features
- Expanded cord

Microscopic Features
- Fibrillary astrocytoma
  - o Increased cellularity, variable atypia/mitoses
  - o Parenchymal infiltration
- Pilocytic astrocytoma
  - o Rosenthal fibers, glomeruloid/hyalinized vessels
  - o Low prevalence of nuclear atypia/mitoses

Staging or Grading Criteria
- 80-90% low grade
  - o Fibrillary astrocytoma = W.H.O. II
  - o Pilocytic astrocytoma = W.H.O. I
  - o Ganglioglioma, mixed gliomas also occur
- 10-15% high grade
  - o Most are anaplastic astrocytomas (W.H.O. III)
  - o Glioblastoma (W.H.O. IV) uncommon

Clinical Issues

Presentation
- Most common initial symptom = back pain
- Symptoms typically evolve over months/years

Natural History
- Most are slow-growing
- Malignant tumors may cause rapid neurologic deterioration

Treatment
- Obtain tissue diagnosis
- Microsurgical resection (low grade tumors)
  - o Intraoperative U/S, evoked potentials helpful
- Adjuvant therapy
  - o No evidence that XRT, chemotherapy improve long-term outcome

Prognosis
- Varies with tumor histology/grade, % gross total resection
  - o 80% 5-year for low grade; 30% for high grade
- Postoperative neurologic function determined largely by degree of preoperative deficit

Selected References
1. Constantini S et al: Radical excision of intramedullary spinal cord tumors: surgical morbidity and long-term follow-up evaluation in 164 children and young adults. J Neurosurg (Spine 2) 93: 183-93, 2000
2. Houten JK et al: Spinal cord astrocytomas: presentation, management and outcome. J Neurooncol 47: 219-4, 2000
3. Minehan KJ et al: Spinal cord astrocytoma: pathological and treatment considerations. J Neurosurg 83: 590-5, 1996

Cord Ependymoma

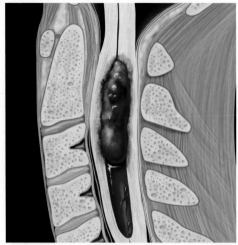

Sagittal graphic depicts an intramedullary ependymoma involving the cervical spinal cord. Note the central location of the tumor, associated neoplastic cyst, and cord expansion. A prominent "cap" of hemosiderin is often seen in these lesions, along with blood products in various stages of degradation.

Key Facts
- Slowly growing cord tumor arising from central canal ependyma
- Most common primary spinal cord tumor in adults
- Second most common primary spinal cord tumor in children
- Associated hemorrhage distinguishes ependymoma from other cord tumors

Imaging Findings
General Features
- Best imaging clue: Circumscribed, enhancing cord mass **with hemorrhage**
- Often multisegmental
- Arises from central canal, causes symmetric cord enlargement
- 50% associated syrinx, "polar" (rostral or caudal) or intratumoral cyst
- May cause nonaneurysmal SAH, superficial siderosis
CT Findings
- NECT
  - May show spinal canal widening
    - Thinned pedicles
    - Widened interpediculate distance
    - Posterior vertebral scalloping
- CECT: Symmetrically enlarged spinal cord + focal enhancement
MR Findings
- T1WI: Isointense to spinal cord (rarely hypointense)
- T2WI
  - Hyperintense
  - Heterogeneous if cyst/hemorrhage
    - "Cap sign" = hypointensity at margin (old hemorrhage)
- Contrast-enhanced T1WI
  - Usually intense, well-delineated homogeneous enhancement

Cord Ependymoma

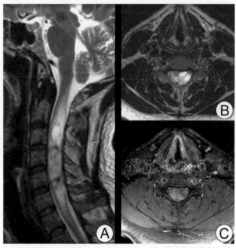

Sagittal and axial T2WI (A, B) and post-contrast axial T1WI (C) show a typical ependymoma. Note central cord expansion and mixed signal intensity caused by blood products. Enhancement degree and pattern is variable in cord ependymomas. Moderate, heterogeneous enhancement is seen in this case.

- o Other: Heterogeneous, rim-like (rare = minimal or no enhancement)

Other Modality Findings
- Myelography/CT myelography
  - o Multisegmental fusiform cord expansion
  - o May cause partial or complete "block"
- Radiography: Scoliosis, canal widening, posterior vertebral body scalloping

Imaging Recommendations
- Contrast-enhanced MR

Differential Diagnosis
Astrocytoma
- May be indistinguishable
- Often longer (can be holocord)
- More often eccentric, infiltrative
- Hemorrhage uncommon

Hemangioblastoma
- Cyst with enhancing highly vascular nodule
- Thoracic > cervical
- Older patients (1/3 have VHL)

Demyelinating Disease (M.S., A.D.E.M.)
- Often multifocal; 90% have brain lesions
- Lesions more often peripheral, posterior/lateral
- Enhancement often faint, poorly marginated ("feathered")

Pathology
General
- General Path Comments
  - o Four subtypes (cellular, papillary, clear-cell, tanycytic)

Cord Ependymoma

- o Cellular most common intramedullary tumor subtype
- o Tumoral and nontumoral cysts (rostral/caudal & syrinx) common
- Genetics
  - o None known for sporadic ependymomas
  - o NF-2-associated ependymoma
    - Deletions, translocations of chromosome 22
- Etiology-Pathogenesis
  - o Arises from ependymal cells of central canal
- Epidemiology
  - o Slight male predominance (57%)
  - o Mean age at presentation = 39y

Gross Pathologic-Surgical Features
- Soft red or grayish-purple mass, often well-circumscribed; cystic degeneration, hemorrhage common

Microscopic Features
- Perivascular pseudorosettes
- True ependymal rosettes (less frequent)
- Moderately cellular with low mitotic activity
- Occasional nuclear atypia, occasional to no mitoses
- Immunohistochemistry: GFAP, S-100, vimentin +

Staging or Grading Criteria
- Most are WHO grade II
- Rare: WHO grade III (anaplastic variant)

Clinical Issues

Presentation
- Most common symptom = pain (neck or back)
- Occasionally sensory or motor complaints predominate
- Often long antecedent history

Natural History
- The less the preoperative neurologic deficit at presentation, the better the postoperative outcome
- Thoracic tumors have worse surgical outcome
- Rarely metastasize (lungs, retroperitoneum, lymph nodes)

Treatment
- Surgical resection
- XRT for subtotal resection or recurrent disease

Prognosis
- 5 year survival 82%

Selected References
1. Wiestler OD et al: Ependymoma. In Kleihues P, Cavanee WK (eds), Pathology & Genetics of Tumours of the Central Nervous System, 72-7. IARC Press, 2000
2. Koeller KK et al: Neoplasms of the spinal cord and filum terminale: Radiologic-pathologic correlation. Radiographics 20: 1721-49, 2000
3. Kahan H et al: MR characteristics of histopathologic subtypes of spinal ependymoma. AJNR 17: 143-50, 1996

Spinal Hemangioblastoma

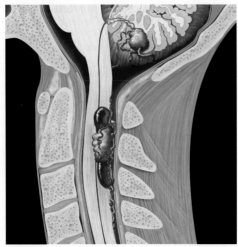

Sagittal graphic depicts vermian, cervical cord hemangioblastomas in a patient with VHL disease. Note subpial location of the vascular tumor nodules. Enlarged feeding arteries and prominent draining veins are common findings. Two small cysts with hemorrhage are associated with the cord lesion.

Key Facts
- Synonym: Capillary hemangioblastoma (HB)
- 1-5% of intramedullary neoplasms
- 75% sporadic; 25% von Hippel-Lindau disease (VHL)
- Multiple tumors (often small) in VHL

Imaging Findings
General Features
- Best imaging clue: Intramedullary mass with serpentine "flow voids"
CT Findings
- NECT: Intramedullary mass +/- expanded/remodeled spinal canal
- CECT: May demonstrate enhancing nodule
MR Findings
- Depend on lesion size, presence of syrinx
- T1WI
  - Small
    - Isointense with cord (may be invisible unless hemorrhage has occurred)
    - Well-delineated syrinx (hypointense) present in > 50%
  - Large
    - Mixed hypo/isointense
    - Lesions =/> 2.5 cm almost always show "flow voids" (enlarged feeding arteries and/or draining veins)
- T2WI (small lesions usually uniformly hyperintense)
  - Mixed hyperintense (flow voids, hemorrhage common)
  - Syrinx fluid often slightly hyperintense to CSF
  - +/- peritumoral edema
- T1WI + contrast
  - Small
    - Subpial nodule (often on surface of dorsal cord)

Spinal Hemangioblastoma

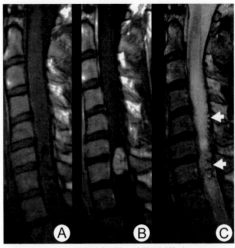

Sagittal pre- and post-contrast T1WI (A, B) and T2WI (C) show an expanded cervical cord with intensely enhancing nodule, extensive edema. Note prominent "flow voids" (arrows). Hemangioblastoma was found at surgery. The patient does not have VHL.

- Well-demarcated, intense, homogeneous enhancement
  o Large
    - Heterogeneous enhancement
    - If syrinx present, wall doesn't enhance

Other Modality Findings
- DSA
  o Enlarged spinal arteries (anterior > posterior) supply mass
  o Intense, prolonged vascular stain
  o +/- A-V shunting

Imaging Recommendations
- Contrast-enhanced MR
  o Scan brain, entire spine in patients with known/suspected VHL!
- DSA for large lesions
- Intraoperative sonography may be useful in locating nodule

Differential Diagnosis
Arteriovenous Malformation (AVM)
- Cord often normal/small, gliotic
- Syrinx, focal nodule absent

Other Hypervascular Cord Neoplasms
- Ependymoma (mass centrally located; no syrinx)
- Vascular metastasis (known primary, e.g., renal cell carcinoma)
- Astrocytoma (usually not hypervascular; peritumoral edema common)
- Paraganglioma (filum >> cord but may be indistinguishable)

Pathology
General
- General Path Comments
  o VHL phenotypes

Spinal Hemangioblastoma

- Type 1 = without pheochromocytoma
- Type 2A = with pheochromocytoma, renal cell carcinoma (RCC)
- Type 2B = with pheochromocytoma, no RCC
- Genetics
  - Familial HB (VHL)
    - Autosomal dominant
    - Chromosome 3p, other gene mutations common
    - VEGF highly expressed
    - Erythropoietin often upregulated
  - Sporadic HB (unknown origin)
- Etiology-Pathogenesis
  - Suppressor gene product (VHL protein) causes neoplastic transformation
- Epidemiology
  - 1-5% of all spinal cord neoplasms
  - 75% of spinal HBs are sporadic (25% VHL-associated)
  - Often multiple (VHL usually has one large +/- many small HBs)

Gross Pathologic-Surgical Features
- Well-circumscribed vascular nodule
  - Dorsal surface of cord
  - Extramedullary spinal HBs occur but are rare
- Prominent arteries, veins
- +/- syrinx

Microscopic Features
- Large vacuolated stromal cells + rich capillary network
- If present, cyst wall usually compressed cord (not tumor)

Staging or Grading Criteria: HBs are WHO grade I!

Clinical Issues

Presentation
- Mean age at presentation = 30y
- Nonspecific clinical symptoms
- Sensory/motor > pain
- VHL patients usually have one dominant symptomatic lesion; may have other smaller, asymptomatic lesions
- May cause secondary polycythemia (erythropoietin upregulated)

Natural History
- Grows slowly
- Does not undergo malignant degeneration

Treatment
- Microsurgical resection

Prognosis
- Life expectancy of VHL patients = 50y
- CNS HBs most common cause of death
- RCCs second

Selected References
1. Chu B-C et al: MR findings in spinal hemangioblastoma: Correlation with symptoms and with angiographic and surgical findings. AJNR 22: 206-17, 2001
2. Baker KB et al: MR imaging of spinal hemangioblastoma. AJR 174: 377-82, 2000
3. Navarra F et al: Spinal cord haemangioblastoma: Epidemiology and neuroradiological diagnosis. Riv di Neuroradiol 9: 289-96, 1996

Aneurysmal Bone Cyst

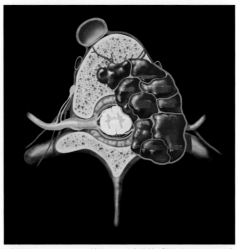

Axial graphic depicts an aneurysmal bone cyst (ABC) of L1. Note expansile, multicystic mass in the posterior vertebral body and pedicle extending into the epidural space. Fluid-fluid levels formed by blood products of different ages are characteristic of ABCs.

Key Facts
- Definition: Expansile lesion with thin-walled, blood-filled, cystic cavities
- 1-2% of bone tumors
- 10-30% in spine/sacrum
- Imaging: Multicystic expansile mass with septations, fluid-fluid levels
- Vast majority < 20y

Imaging Findings
General Features
- Best imaging clue: Expansile multiloculated neural arch mass with fluid-fluid levels
  - Extension into vertebral bodies, canal, epidural space common
  - Involvement of ribs, paraspinal soft tissues less common
  - Rare: Crosses disc space, involves > 1 vertebra (only benign bone tumor that does)
CT Findings
- NECT
  - Expansile, cystic, septated mass with intact thin "eggshell" cortex
  - Fluid-fluid levels caused by hemorrhage, blood product sedimentation
- CECT: Periphery, septa enhance
MR Findings
- T1WI
  - Lobulated multicystic neural arch mass
    - Extends into vertebral body +/- adjacent soft tissue
    - Mixed intensity, fluid-fluid levels (blood products)
  - Hypointense rim (periosteal membrane)
- T2WI
  - Intensities vary with stage of blood degradation
  - Hypointense rim (periosteal membrane)
- Contrast-enhanced T1WI

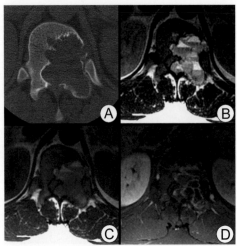

A 19-year-old male with low back pain. NECT (A) shows an expansile mass with thin "eggshell" cortex. Axial T2-, pre- and post-contrast T1WI (B, C, D) show the septated mass with fluid-fluid levels and mixed signal intensity related to blood products of varying ages. Note enhancement of septations. ABC.

- o Rim, septa enhance

<u>Other Modality Findings</u>
- Radiography
  - o Marked expansile remodeling of bone
    - Epicenter in posterior elements with extension into vertebral body (75-90%)
    - Thin outer periosteal rim and septations may be seen
    - Rare: Vertebral body collapse ("vertebra plana")
- Radionuclide scan: Peripheral increased uptake ("donut sign")
- DSA: Hypervascular

<u>Imaging Recommendations</u>
- MRI for epidural extent, cord compromise
- CT for bone changes

Differential Diagnosis
<u>Osteoblastoma</u>
- Expansile lesion of neural arch/pedicle > 2 cm

<u>Metastases</u>
- Older patients (usually 6th, 7th decades)
- Destructive lesion with associated soft-tissue mass
- Rare: Vascular metastasis can have fluid levels

<u>Giant Cell Tumor</u>
- Patients > 30y
- Expansile, lytic lesion with associated soft-tissue mass

Pathology
<u>General</u>
- General Path Comments
  - o Location

Aneurysmal Bone Cyst

- Long bone metaphysis > vertebra
- Thoracic > Lumbar > Cervical >> Sacrum
- Most common - posterior elements alone or + vertebral body
- o Characteristic multiloculated blood-filled spaces
- Etiology-Pathogenesis
  - o 2 theories
    - 1°: Results from trauma + local circulatory disturbance
    - 2°: Underlying tumor (GCT, OB, etc) induces vascular process (venous obstruction or AV fistulae)
- Epidemiology
  - o 1-2% of primary bone tumors
  - o 10-30% occur in axial skeleton
  - o Majority of ABCs are primary lesions (65-99%)
  - o 80% are < 20y
  - o Slight female predominance

Microscopic Features
- Typical
  - o Cystic component predominates
    - Cavernous blood-filled cysts of variable sizes
    - Lined by fibroblasts, giant cells, histiocytes, hemosiderin
  - o Solid components
    - Septations interposed between blood-filled spaces
    - Contain fibrous tissue, reactive bone, giant cells
- Rare = "solid variant"
  - o Only 5-8% of all ABCs
  - o Solid component predominates
  - o Propensity for spine

Clinical Issues

Presentation
- Most common = pain
- Less common = neurologic symptoms (cord compression, pathologic fx)

Natural History
- Long-term history of untreated ABC unknown
  - o Grows initially, then usually stabilizes
  - o No malignant degeneration

Treatment
- Surgical excision
- Embolization (preoperative or for poor surgical candidates)
- XRT controversial (may predispose to radiation-induced sarcoma)

Prognosis
- Recurrence rate 20-30% (increased if incomplete excision)

Selected References
1. Papagelopoulos PJ et al: Aneurysmal bone cyst of the spine: Management and outcome. Spine 23: 621-8, 1998
2. Murphey MD et al: Primary tumors of the spine: Radiologic-pathologic correlation. RadioGraphics 16:1131-58, 1996
3. Kransdorf MJ et al: Aneurysmal bone cyst: Concept, controversy, clinical presentation, and imaging. AJR 164: 573-80, 1995

Langerhans Cell Histiocytosis

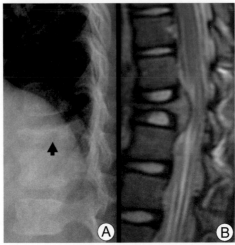

Lateral plain film (A) in a 4 yo male with back pain shows vertebra plana (arrow). Sagittal T2WI (B) in a 5 yo male with LCH shows a collapsed vertebral body with normal adjacent discs. Note posterior epidural extension, common for LCH.

Key Facts
- Synonyms: Eosinophilic granuloma (EG), histiocytosis X, LCH
- Definition: Collection(s) of abnormal histiocytes (Langerhans cells)
- 3 clinical syndromes recognized
  - EG (70% of LCH)
    - Localized form (bone lesions only)
    - Older children (5-15y)
  - Hand-Schuller-Christian disease (20% of LCH)
    - Chronic disseminated form
    - Younger children (1-5y)
  - Letterer-Siwe disease (10% of LCH)
    - Acute disseminated form
    - Infants (<3y)
- Imaging: Lytic and/or collapsed vertebral body (vertebra plana)

Imaging Findings
General Features
- Best imaging clue: Child with vertebra plana
  - Two apposed intervertebral discs (looks like no intervening vertebral body is present) (adjacent discs may appear enlarged)
  - Associated soft tissue mass common (+/- extends into spinal canal)
CT Findings
- NECT
  - Lytic, destructive lesion without sclerosis
  - Vertebra plana +/- soft tissue mass
- CECT: Soft tissue mass enhances homogeneously
MR Findings
- T1WI: Hypointense vertebral body, soft tissue mass
- T2WI: Heterogeneously hyperintense
- T1WI with contrast: Homogeneous enhancement

Langerhans Cell Histiocytosis

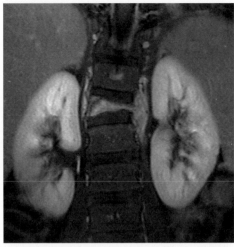

Coronal post-contrast T1WI from same case as (B) on previous page shows homogenous enhancement. Note scoliosis and paraspinal soft tissue mass.

Other Modality Findings
- Radiography
  - Collapsed vertebral body, normal adjacent discs
  - Rare: Posterior elements involved
- Radionuclide scans: Variable (increased uptake typical); false negative common (35%)

Imaging Recommendations
- MRI to evaluate spinal canal

Differential Diagnosis

Ewing Sarcoma
- Permeative bone destruction

Osteomyelitis
- Hyperintense narrowed disc

Metastases, Neuroblastoma, Hemopoietic Disorders (leukemia/lymphoma)
- Multifocal disease, often associated soft tissue component
- May be indistinguishable from LCH

Giant Cell Tumor
- Older patients (>30y)
- Expansile, lytic vertebral lesion + soft tissue mass
- May extend to posterior elements; may present as vertebra plana

Pathology

General
- General Path Comments
  - Location
    - Calvarium > mandible > long bones > ribs > pelvis > vertebrae
    - Thoracic (54%) > lumbar (35%) > cervical (11%)

Langerhans Cell Histiocytosis

- Etiology-Pathogenesis
  - o Disorder of immune regulation
  - o Proliferation of abnormal histiocytes
  - o Reticuloendothelial system (RES) forms granulomas
- Epidemiology
  - o < 1% of biopsy-proven primary bone lesions
  - o 0.05-0.5 per 100,000 children per year
  - o Slight male predominance
  - o Vertebral involvement 6%
  - o Most common cause of vertebra plana in children

<u>Gross Pathologic-Surgical Features</u>
- Yellow, grey, or brown mass, +/- hemorrhage

<u>Microscopic Features</u>
- Light microscopy shows granulomatous infiltrates
  - o Langerhans cell histiocytes, macrophages
  - o Lymphocytes, plasma cells, eosinophils
- EM: Birbeck granules (Langerhans cell granules)

Clinical Issues

<u>Presentation</u>
- 3 clinical syndromes recognized in LCH
  - o EG (70%), peak = 5-15y
    - ▪ Mildest form, affects single or multiple bones
    - ▪ Local pain, swelling, mass, +/- fever and leukocytosis
    - ▪ Spine - back pain, stiffness, scoliosis, neurologic complications
  - o Hand-Schuller-Christian disease (20%), peak = 1-5y
    - ▪ Most varied, chronic dissemination of osseous lesions
    - ▪ Triad of diabetes insipidus, exophthalmos, bone destruction (15%)
    - ▪ Clinical: Skull involvement >90%; other = otitis media, cutaneous involvement, gum ulceration, lymphadenopathy, hepatosplenomegaly
    - ▪ Fatal 10-30%
  - o Letterer-Siwe disease (10%), usually <3y
    - ▪ Acute form, rapid dissemination, poor prognosis
    - ▪ Multiple visceral organs involved; fevers, cachexia, anemia, hepatosplenomegaly, lymphadenopathy, rash, gum hyperplasia
    - ▪ Calvarium, skull base, mandible most often involved
    - ▪ Most patients die within 1-2 years

<u>Natural History</u>
- Varies with clinical type
- EG self-limited; some restoration of vertebral height

<u>Treatment</u>
- Conservative management
- +/- Surgical intervention, XRT, chemotherapy, steroids

<u>Prognosis</u>
- Dependent on age at presentation, type/extent of systemic disease
- EG has best prognosis; spontaneous remission of lesions typical

Selected References
1. Yeom JS et al: Langerhans' cell histiocytosis of the spine. Analysis of twenty-three cases. Spine 24: 1740-9, 1999
2. Meyer JS et al: Langerhans cell histiocytosis: Presentation and evolution of radiologic findings with clinical correlation. RadioGraphics 15: 1135-46, 1995
3. Stull MA et al: Langerhans cell histiocytosis of bone. RadioGraphics 12: 801-23, 1992

NON-NEOPLASTIC CYSTS AND MASSES

Spinal Arachnoid Cyst

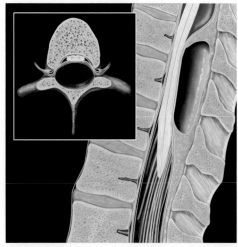

Sagittal illustration of the lumbosacral spine demonstrates a posterior epidural arachnoid cyst (Type I meningeal cyst), compressing the thecal sac. The cyst is "capped" by epidural fat cranially and caudally. Axial inset demonstrates its epidural location and mass effect on the thecal sac.

Key Facts

- Synonym: Spinal meningeal cyst (MC)
- Definition: Intraspinal extramedullary cerebral spinal fluid (CSF) containing cyst
- Classic imaging appearance
  - Intradural or extradural
  - CSF intensity on all pulse sequences
  - Variable mass effect on the spinal cord or the thecal sac
- Other key facts
  - Primary or congenital vs secondary or acquired
  - Acquired intradural arachnoid cyst (AC) also known as subarachnoid cyst
  - Nabors classification of spinal MC
  - Type I: Extradural MC without spinal nerve root fibers
    - Also known as extradural AC
    - Relatively rare
    - Primary extradural AC usually in the posterior or posterolateral aspect of the lower thoracic spine
    - May extend into neural foramina
  - Type II: Extradural MC with spinal nerve root fibers
    - Includes perineural root sleeve (Tarlov) cyst
  - Type III: Intradural MC
    - Also known as intradural AC
    - Primary intradural AC commonly in the posterior aspect of the midthoracic spine
    - Secondary intradural AC without specific location
  - MRI is the imaging modality of choice

Spinal Arachnoid Cyst

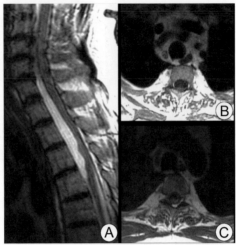

Sagittal T2WI (A) demonstrates an anterior intraspinal fluid intensity lesion, extending from C6 to T4. It displaces the spinal cord posteriorly, producing a scalloped appearance on the ventral surface of the cord. Axial T1WI (B, C) at two different levels confirm its intradural location.

Imaging Findings

<u>General Features</u>
- Best imaging clue: Asymmetric, loculated CSF intensity collection displacing or deforming the cord or nerve roots

<u>Myelography Findings</u>
- Intradural or extradural mass
- Spinal cord compression
- Complete myelographic block
- Filling of AC
  - Sometimes on delayed imaging

<u>Postmyelography CT Findings</u>
- Same as above
- Spinal canal enlargement
- Neural foraminal extension and enlargement
- Thinned pedicles and laminae if long-standing (congenital)

<u>Plain Film Findings</u>
- Posterior vertebral body scalloping

<u>MR Findings</u>
- Extradural or intradural extramedullary mass
- CSF intensity on all pulse sequences
  - Hypointensity on T2WI may be related to flow related signal loss
- Cyst wall may be imperceptible
- Solitary, multiple, or multiloculated
- Extradural AC may extend through enlarged neural foramina
- No post-gadolinium enhancement
- Variable mass effect on the spinal cord
- Associated spinal cord myelomalacia
- Associated syringohydromyelia at or away from the site of the AC

Spinal Arachnoid Cyst

Differential Diagnosis
Dural Ectasia Associated with Marfan's Syndrome or Other Causes
- Diffuse dilatation of the thecal sac
- Spinal cord not distorted
- No block on myelogram or CT myelogram

Spinal Nerve Root Avulsion
- Contiguous with the subarachnoid space
- No discrete intraspinal lesion
- History of trauma

Pathology
General
- Etiology-Pathogenesis
  - Primary intradural AC thought to arise from diverticulum of the arachnoid matter
  - Primary extradural AC thought to arise from arachnoid protrusion through a dural defect
    - Both may or may not communicate with the arachnoid space through a neck
    - Enlargement possibly due to "ball valve" mechanism
  - Secondary AC result from prior trauma, surgery, infection, or hemorrhage
    - Posttraumatic dural tear with arachnoid herniation
    - Post-inflammatory granulation tissue may compartmentalize the subarachnoid space
    - Subsequent cyst development

Microscopic Features
- Primary AC usually lined with arachnoid matter, sometimes duplicated
- Variable connective tissue also forming the cyst wall

Clinical Issues
Presentation
- Pain
- Weakness
- Sensory level
- Radicular symptoms

Natural History
- Worsening neurological deficits with enlarging cyst

Treatment
- Surgical resection
- Marsupialization of the cyst
- Shunting

Prognosis
- Excellent, with relief of symptoms
- Degree of cord atrophy predictive of neurological outcome

Selected References
1. Silbergleit R et al: Imaging of spinal intradural arachnoid cysts: MRI, myelography and CT. Neuroradiology 40:664-8, 1998
2. Sklar E et al: Acquired spinal subarachnoid cysts: Evaluation with MR, CT myelography, and intraoperative sonography. AJNR 10:1097-104, 1989
3. Gray L et al: MR imaging of thoracic extradural arachnoid cysts. JACT 4:664-8, 1988

Posterior Sacral Meningocele

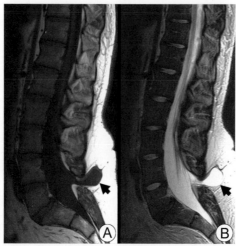

Sagittal T1- (A), T2WIs (B) demonstrate a posterior sacral meningocele at the level of L4-5 (arrows). The filum terminale appears thickened, tethered into the neck of the herniation sac. A small focal fatty element is seen and the distal spinal canal is expanded.

Key Facts
- Definition: Herniation of cerebral spinal fluid (CSF)-containing sac lined by dura and arachnoid, through a bony defect in the sacrum
- Classic imaging appearance: Focal posterior outpouching of the thecal sac through a spina bifida defect
- Covered by skin
- Does not contain neural elements
  - Most common of all simple meningoceles
  - Lumbosacral > cervical or thoracic
  - Spina bifida in one or two segments
  - Nerve root may enter and then exit the meningocele before leaving the neural foramen
  - Filum terminale may extend into the sac
  - May have associated occult spinal anomalies
    - Low lying conus, tight filum, split cord malformation, epidermoid, dorsal lipoma, and hydromyelia
- Other simple meningoceles
  - Anterior sacral meningocele
    - Associated with anorectal malformation and sacral anomalies
    - Currarino's triad
  - Distal sacral or intrasacral meningocele
    - Also known as type IB meningeal cyst
  - Lateral thoracic meningocele
    - Commonly seen in patients with neurofibromatosis, type I

Imaging Findings
<u>General Features</u>
- Best imaging clue: Communicates with the subarachnoid space

Posterior Sacral Meningocele

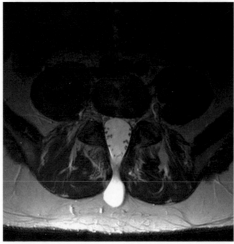

In addition to the meningocele, axial T2WI reveals a spina bifida defect.

CT Findings
- CSF density thin walled collection
- Variable extension into the posterior subcutaneous soft tissue
- Spectrum of bony abnormality
  - Absent single spinous process
  - Single level spina bifida
  - Multisegmental spina bifida
- Spinal canal may be enlarged

MR Findings
- Same intensity as CSF on all sequences
- No postgadolinium enhancement
- Low lying conus and causes of tethering may be present

Ultrasound Findings
- Posterior anechoic sac contiguous with the thecal sac
- Changes size with Valsalva maneuver

Imaging Recommendations
- Careful evaluation of the spinal cord to exclude associated anomalies

Differential Diagnosis

Myelomeningocele
- Neural elements within the meningocele
- Protruding beyond the sacral soft tissue
- Not covered by skin
- Discovered at birth

Lipomyelomeningocele
- Lipoma-neural placode complex within the meningocele
- Covered by skin

Post-surgical Meningocele
- Same appearance
- History and findings of laminectomy

Posterior Sacral Meningocele

Pathology

General

- Etiology-Pathogenesis
  - Unknown
- Epidemiology
  - Usually presents in the first two decades of life
  - May present as late as the fourth decade
  - M:F = 1:1

Clinical Issues

Presentation

- If large, may see a posterior lumbosacral contour bulge
- Subcutaneous mass may be palpable
- Neurological symptoms if cord tethered

Treatment

- Surgical resection
- Closure of the dura

Prognosis

- Good
- Post-surgical scarring may tether the cord
  - Presenting as a complication later in life

Selected References

1. Ersahin Y et al: Is meningocele really an isolated lesion? Childs Nerv Syst 17:487-90, 2001
2. Barkovich AJ: Pediatric Neuroimaging. 2nd ed. 491-496, 1995
3. Byrd SE et al: Developmental disorders of the pediatric spine. Radiol Clin North Am 29:711-52, 1991

Epidermoid Tumor

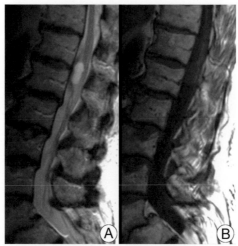

Sagittal T2WI (A) and T1WI (B) of the lumbar spine in an older patient demonstrate an ovoid intraspinal lesion adherent to the conus medullaris. Compared to CSF, it is hyperintense on T2WI and slightly hyperintense on T1WI.

Key Facts
- Synonym: (Epi)dermoid cyst
- Definition: Congenital or acquired intraspinal tumors arising from inclusion of (ecto)dermal elements
- Classic imaging appearance: Nonenhancing fat intensity (dermoid) or CSF intensity (epidermoid) mass
- Congenital lesions
  - 1% to 2% of spinal tumors
  - 60% extramedullary and 40% intramedullary
  - Dermoids occur more commonly in the spine compared to epidermoids
    - Most common in the lumbosacral region
    - Symptomatic before the second decade of life
  - Epidermoids evenly distributed throughout the spine
    - Symptomatic around the third to fifth decades of life
  - 20% of (epi)dermoids associated with dermal sinus
    - May present with meningitis or spinal abscess
  - (Epi)dermoids may rupture and produce chemical meningitis
- Acquired lesions
  - Extramedullary
    - Adherent to the spinal cord, cauda equina, or the thecal sac
  - Occur after surgical repair of myelomeningocele or remote lumbar puncture

Imaging Findings
General Features
- Best imaging clue: Fat intensity (dermoid), or CSF intensity (epidermoid)
CT Myelogram Findings
- Intra- or extramedullary hypodense lesion
- Myelographic block may be present with large extramedullary lesion

Epidermoid Tumor

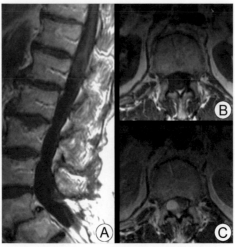

Post-contrast sagittal T1WI (A) in a patient with back pain shows a questionable lesion adjacent to the conus medullaris. The lesion is nearly isointense with CSF on axial T1WI (B). (C) Long TR/short TE scan shows the lesion well and confirms its intradural extramedullary location. Epidermoid was found at surgery.

MR Findings
- Dermoids
  - Hyperintense on T1WI (fat intensity)
    - May have low to intermediate signal intensity, between CSF and cord
  - Hyperintense on T2WI
- Epidermoids
  - Similar or isointense to CSF on T1WI
    - May be isointense to cord
  - Iso- to hyperintense to CSF on T2WI
- No post-gadolinium enhancement
- CSF-isointense extramedullary lesion can be very subtle
  - May be suggested by nerve root or cord displacement
- Chemical arachnoiditis from ruptured (epi)dermoid
- Intra- or extramedullary abscess may be seen with dermal sinus
- Abscess and arachnoiditis best seen with gadolinium on T1WI

Imaging Recommendations
- Heavily T1-weighted sequence (inversion recovery or SPGR) may distinguish subtle extramedullary masses from CSF
- CT myelography can also supplement MR in delineating extramedullary CSF-isointense masses

Differential Diagnosis

Intraspinal Neoplasm
- Isointense to cord on T1WI
- Hyperintense on T2WI
- Intramedullary mass with peritumoral edema
- Postgadolinium enhancement

- Carcinomatous meningitis may show diffuse and sheet-like or focal and nodular enhancement

Intraspinal Lipoma
- Hyperintense mass on T1WI
- Fades on late-echo T2WI or with fat saturation
- Typically midline
- Very smooth margins

Pathology
General
- Embryology-Anatomy
  - o The neural tube forms by the infolding and closure of the neural ectoderm
    - As it separates from the cutaneous ectoderm
    - Occurring in the third and fourth week of the embryonic life
    - In a process known as neurulation and disjunction
- Etiology-Pathogenesis
  - o Congenital lesions result from focal incorporation of the cutaneous ectoderm into the neural ectoderm during disjunction
  - o Acquired lesions occur as (ecto)dermal elements iatrogenically introduced into the thecal sac during lumbar puncture or dysraphism repair
- Epidemiology
  - o Congenital lesions
    - Dermoid equally common in males and females
    - Epidermoid more common in males

Gross Pathologic-Surgical Features
- Discrete pearly white tumors
- May see cheesy, oily material in dermoids

Microscopic Features
- Desquamated epithelium with solid crystalline cholesterol in epidermoids
- Skin adnexa (sebaceous glands, blood vessels, and hair follicles) in dermoids

Clinical Issues
Presentation
- Meningitis or spinal abscess when dermal sinus present
- Chemical arachnoiditis from ruptured (epi)dermoids
- Enlarging tumor causes myelopathy
  - o Back and lower extremity pain
  - o Paraparesis
  - o Sensory disturbance
  - o Sphincter dysfunction

Treatment
- Surgical resection

Prognosis
- Surgery curative
- Neurological sequelae associated with tethered cord or myelomeningocele

Selected References
1. Barkovich AJ: Pediatric Neuroimaging. 2nd ed. 491-6, 1995
2. Gupta S et al: Signal intensity patterns in intraspinal dermoids and epidermoids on MR imaging. Clin Radiol 48:405-13, 1993
3. Toro VE et al: MRI of iatrogenic spinal epidermoid tumor. JACT 17:970-2, 1993

Spinal Epidural Lipomatosis

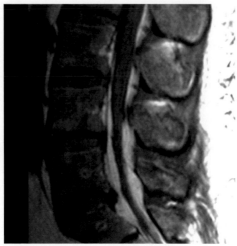

Unenhanced sagittal T1WI shows increased fat within the distal spinal canal, surrounding the thecal sac.

Key Facts
- Excessive epidural fat surrounding the thoracic and lumbar thecal sac

Imaging Findings
General Features
- Best imaging clue: Abundant fat tissue in the spinal canal
  - Tapering of the thecal sac
  - Crowding of the cauda equina

CT Findings
- Increased fat density in the distal spinal canal
- Narrowing of the thecal sac

MR Findings
- Modality of choice for visualization of fat
- Homogeneous and hyperintense on both T1-weighted and T2-weighted sequences
- Hypointense on fat-suppressed imaging
- Mass effect on the thecal sac and nerve roots
- Scalloped appearance to the thecal sac

Differential Diagnosis
Subacute Hemorrhage in Sudural or Epidural Space
- Fat saturation can help distinguish fat from hemorrhage

Pathology
General
- General Path Comments
  - Increased fat tissue in the spinal canal
  - Typically in the thoracic and lumbar regions
- Etiology-Pathogenesis
  - Exogenous steroid administration
  - Excessive endogenous steroid production

Spinal Epidural Lipomatosis

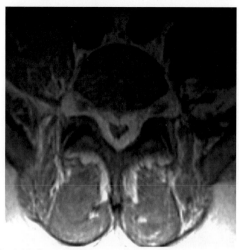

Axial T1WI at L4-5 demonstrates increased epidural fat compressing the thecal sac and surrounding the nerve roots.

- o General obesity
- o Idiopathic

Gross Pathologic-Surgical Features
- Abundant fat tissue external to the thecal sac

Microscopic Features
- Hypertrophied fat cells

Clinical Issues

Presentation
- Principal presenting symptom: Chronic back pain
- Polyradiculopathy
- Myelopathy
- Neurogenic claudication

Treatment
- Correction of underlying endocrinopathies
- Dieting in the case of general obesity
- Surgical intervention
  - o Multilevel laminectomy
  - o Fat debulking
  - o Posterolateral fusion

Prognosis
- Excellent

Selected References
1. Lisai P et al: Cauda Equina Syndrome Secondary to Idiopathic Spinal Epidural Lipomatosis. Spine Vol 26:307-9, 2001
2. Kumar K et al: Symptomatic Epidural lipomatosis Secondary to Obesity. J Neurosurg Vol 85: 348-50, 1996

Type II Meningeal Cyst

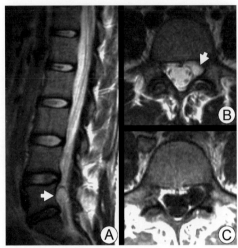

Sagittal T2WI (A) of the lumbar spine demonstrates a circumscribed intraspinal CSF intensity cyst (arrow) at the level of L5. Axial T2WI (B) shows this cyst (arrow) to be in the left lateral recess, contacting the thecal sac. There is no enhancement after intravenous gadolinium on T1WI(C).

Key Facts

- Synonyms: Perineural cyst, spinal nerve root diverticulum, also known as Tarlov's cyst in the sacrum
- Definition: Congenital dilatation of the arachnoid and dura composing the spinal nerve root sleeve
- Classic imaging appearance: Cerebral spinal fluid (CSF) intensity cyst(s) enlarging the sacral foramina
- Other key facts
  - Nabors classification of congenital spinal Meningeal cyst (MC) based on operative findings
  - Type I: Extradural MC without spinal nerve root fibers
    - IA: Extradural MC, also known as extradural arachnoid cyst
    - Relatively rare
    - Usually in the posterior or posterolateral aspect of the lower thoracic spine
    - May extend into neural foramina
    - IB: Sacral meningocele
    - Connected to the caudal tip of thecal sac by a pedicle
  - Type II: Extradural MC with spinal nerve root fibers
    - Anywhere along the spine, more common in the lower lumbar spine and the sacrum
    - Multiple and bilateral, some larger than others
    - Common, incidental, and usually asymptomatic, rare cause of sciatica
    - No reliable imaging method to differentiate symptomatic from asymptomatic lesions
  - Type III: Intradural MC
    - Also known as intradural arachnoid cyst
    - Commonly in the posterior aspect of the midthoracic spine

Type II Meningeal Cyst

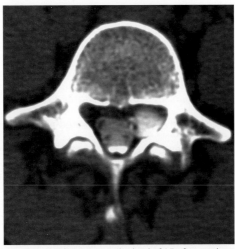

Axial CT image of the lumbar spine at the level of L5 after myelography reveals opacification of the meningeal cyst by intrathecal contrast, suggesting communication with the subarachnoid space.

Imaging Findings
General Features
- Best imaging clue: Intraspinal mass with CSF intensity on all MR sequences

CT Findings
- CSF density cyst(s)
- Widened canal, enlarged foramina, thinned pedicles, and scalloped vertebral bodies or sacrum

MR Findings
- No post-gadolinium enhancement
- Flow sensitive sequence may demonstrate signal loss within the cyst, possibly due to inflow of CSF from the subarachnoid space

CT Myelogram Findings
- Opacification of MC by intrathecal contrast, sometimes on delayed imaging

Differential Diagnosis
Spinal Nerve Root Avulsion (Pseudomeningocele)
- Usually unilateral and at contiguous levels
- More common in the lower cervical and upper thoracic spine
- No bony erosion
- History of trauma

Sacral Meningocele
- Large, solitary, CSF-intensity cyst filling most of the sacral canal
- Nerve roots displaced around the cyst
- No neural foraminal extension or bony erosion

Type II Meningeal Cyst

Pathology
General
- Etiology-Pathogenesis
  - Congenital arachnoid proliferation within the root sleeve, versus
  - Posttraumatic rupture of the perineurium and epineurium, leading to cyst formation
    - Common pathway of stenotic cyst ostium
    - Valve-like mechanism allowing pulsatile CSF inflow, limiting egress
- Epidemiology
  - 4.6% in 500 consecutive patients examined with lumbar MRI

Gross Pathologic-Surgical Features
- Originating at the junction of the dorsal nerve root and the dorsal nerve root ganglion
- Spinal nerve roots traversing through the cyst or within the cyst wall

Microscopic Features
- Outer wall with epineurium lined by arachnoid
- Inner wall lined with pia mater

Clinical Issues
Presentation
- Incidental finding
- Low back and leg pain
- Lower extremity numbness
- Bladder or bowel dysfunction

Treatment
- Temporary relief with cyst aspiration
- Partial resection with oversewing of the cyst wall
- Complete resection, sacrificing the nerve root

Prognosis
- Cyst may reinflate following aspiration or partial resection
- Neurologic deficit following complete excision

Selected References
1. Paulsen RD et al: Prevalence and percutaneous drainage of cysts of the sacral nerve root sheath (Tarlov cysts). AJNR 15:293-7, 1994
2. Davis SW et al: Sacral meningeal cysts: Evaluation with MR imaging. Radiology 187:445-8, 1993
3. Nabors MW et al: Updated assessment and current classification of spinal meningeal cysts. J Neurosurg 68:366-77, 1988

POST OPERATIVE COMPLICATIONS

Pseudomeningocele

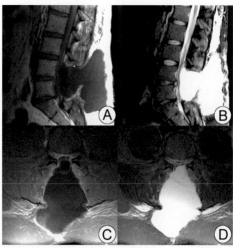

Postoperative pseudomeningocele. (A,B) Sagittal T1WI and FSEIR images show large CSF cyst at surgical site extending dorsally from dural sac into subcutaneous tissues. (C,D) Axial fat saturated T1WI post contrast and T2WI confirm cyst extension through laminectomy and contiguity with thecal sac defect.

Key Facts
- Synonym(s): Dural dehiscence, pseudocyst
- Definition: Spinal cyst that is unlined by meninges and contiguous with thecal sac
- Classic imaging appearance: CSF signal/density collection contiguous with thecal sac in correct clinical context
- Usually posttraumatic or postoperative complication
  - Posttraumatic pseudomeningoceles usually devoid of neural elements
    - May see cord or nerve herniation with severe dural laceration
  - Postoperative pseudomeningocele may contain neural elements

Imaging Findings
General Features
- Best imaging clue: CSF filled spinal axis cyst with supportive post-operative or post-traumatic ancillary findings
CT Findings
- CSF density cyst
- Cervical root avulsions are anterolaterally oriented and contiguous with neural foramen; devoid of neural elements
- Postoperative pseudomeningocele cyst is oriented along operative approach
  - May contain herniated neural elements
  - Dural connection is difficult to demonstrate without intrathecal contrast
MR Findings
- CSF signal intensity cyst
- In postoperative cases, can frequently can identify the thecal sac communication using axial and sagittal T2 weighted imaging
- Does not enhance unless inflamed or infected; may see thin peripheral enhancement within 1 year of surgery

Pseudomeningocele

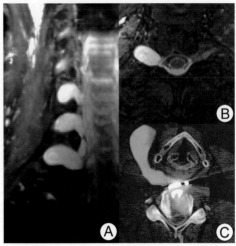

Posttraumatic pseudomeningocele.(A) Coronal FSEIR shows C5, C6, and C7 root avulsions/pseudomeningoceles. Unusual cord appearance is post-processing artifact. (B) Axial FSIER confirms absence of neural elements. Post-operative leak. (C) Axial CT myelogram shows contrast leak at fusion level in different patient.

- Spinal and intracranial dural thickening and enhancement in patients with symptomatic CSF hypotension

Other Modality Findings
- Ultrasound – hypoechoic cyst; difficult to avoid bone shadow in adults

Imaging Recommendations
- Fat saturated T2WI or FSEIR are the best sequences to demonstrate pseudomeningocele and to localize dural communication
- Sagittal plane useful for diagnosis and to tailor thin section axial imaging for definitive localization

Differential Diagnosis

True Meningocele
- Neurofibromatosis type 1, Marfan's syndrome, homocystinuria, and Ehlers-Danlos syndrome
- Does not have pertinent trauma or surgical history
- Often co-exists with dural dysplasia

Plexiform Neurofibroma
- T2 hyperintense
  - Neurofibroma is not as bright as CSF
- Avid contrast enhancement

Pathology

General
- Genearl Path Comments
  - CSF – containing cyst in contiguity with thecal sac
  - Not lined by meninges
  - Usually devoid of neural elements
  - In some cases neural elements may herniate into defect

Pseudomeningocele

- Etiology-Pathogenesis
  - o Posttraumatic
    - Most commonly following cervical root avulsion
    - May also see with posterior element fractures and dural laceration
  - o Post–surgical
    - Iatrogenic dural laceration with CSF leak
    - May also see after dural graft following spinal tumor resection

Microscopic Features
- No meningeal covering

Clinical Issues

Presentation
- Palpable mass, back pain, headache (CSF hypotension), infection

Treatment
- Closure of underlying dural defect when possible
  - o Surgical repair for large defects
  - o Blood patch may be effective for small defects

Prognosis
- Cervical root avulsion usually leaves permanent neurological deficits
- Postoperative defects may close spontaneously if small, but often require treatment

Selected References
1. Bosacco SJ et al: Evaluation and treatment of dural tears in lumbar spine surgery: a review. Clin Orthop 389: 238-47, 2001
2. Jinkins JR et al: The postsurgical lumbosacral spine. Magnetic resonance imaging evaluation following intervertebral disk surgery, surgical decompression, intervertebral bony fusion, and spinal instrumentation. Radiol clin North Am 39(1): 1-29, 2001
3. Ross JS: Magnetic resonance imaging of the postoperative spine. Semin Musculoskelet Radiol 4(3): 281-91, 2000

CSF Leakage Syndromes

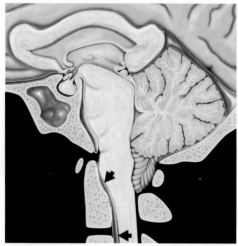

Sagittal graphic depicts the "slumping" midbrain, tonsillar herniation (sometimes called "acquired Chiari I"), and engorged dura (arrows) characteristic for intracranial hypotension. In some cases the spinal epidural venous plexus becomes massively enlarged (see illustration on next page).

Key Facts

- Synonym(s): Spontaneous intracranial hypotension (SIH)
- Reduced CSF pressure with compensatory venous engorgement
- Classic imaging appearance (spine): Thick dura and/or giant epidural veins +/- extradural/paraspinous CSF collection
- Can be spontaneous, traumatic, iatrogenic (post-LP, surgery)
- 20% of spontaneous CSF leaks have minor skeletal features of Marfan

Imaging Findings

General Features

- Best imaging clue: Dural thickening and/or markedly enlarged epidural veins + CSF fluid collection

CT Findings

- NECT
  - Symmetric anterolateral epidural masses (dilated epidural veins)
  - +/- CSF collection (ventral sub/epidural or paraspinous)
  - +/- arachnoid diverticula/meningocele(s)
- CECT
  - May see "draped curtain" sign (intensely enhancing epidural veins)

MR Findings

- T1WI
  - Ventral/anterolateral fluid isointense with CSF, +/- "flow voids"
- T2WI
  - Extra-axial fluid like CSF (may be hyperintense on PD)
  - +/- arachnoid diverticulae
- Contrast-enhanced T1WI
  - Intensely enhancing, greatly enlarged venous plexi
  - Variable dural thickening, enhancement
- MR "myelography" (STIR, fat-suppressed T2WI)
  - Arachnoid diverticulae (often multiple)

CSF Leakage Syndromes

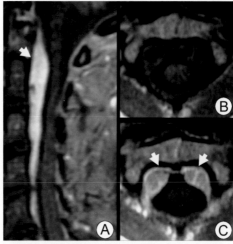

Sagittal post-contrast T1WI (A) and axial pre- (B) and post-contrast (C) scans in a patient with CSF leak and intracranial hypotension show an unusually prominent cervical epidural venous plexus. Note "draped curtain" appearance and prominent flow voids on axial images (case courtesy G. Williams).

- o May demonstrate CSF leak

Other Modality Findings
- Isotope cisternography
  - o Rapid clearance ("washout") from CSF space
  - o Early appearance of radionuclide in kidneys, bladder common
  - o 60% demonstrate CSF leak
- Myelography/CT myelography
  - o Arachnoid diverticula
  - o May demonstrate CSF leak

Imaging Recommendations
- Scan the brain first (look for cranial findings of SIH)
  - o Dural thickening, enhancement
  - o "Sagging midbrain"
  - o Tonsillar herniation
  - o Subdural hygroma
  - o Caution: Not all cases have all classic findings!
- Scan spine, search for actual leakage site only
  - o If two technically adequate blood patches fail
  - o Posttraumatic leak suspected

Differential Diagnosis
Other Causes of Enlarged Spinal Venous Plexi
- AVM
- Jugular vein thrombosis (collateral drainage)
- Venous engorgement above high grade spinal stenosis

Pachymeningopathies
- Infection
  - o Epidural abscess
  - o Rarely occurs in absence of bone, disc involvement

CSF Leakage Syndromes

- Neoplasm (posterior cortex, pedicle often destroyed/infiltrated)
- Miscellaneous (e.g., sarcoid)

Pathology
General
- General Path Comments
  o Usually unremarkable
- Etiology = reduced CSF pressure precipitated by
  o Surgery or trauma (including trivial fall)
  o Vigorous exercise, violent coughing
  o After lumbar puncture
  o Abnormal dura (e.g., Marfan syndrome)
  o Ruptured arachnoid diverticulum
  o Severe dehydration
- Epidemiology
  o F:M = 2:1 (spontaneous)
  o Peak age = 30-40y

Gross Pathologic-Surgical Features
- Engorged cervical epidural veins

Microscopic Features
- Thick dura with fibrosis, numerous dilated thin-walled vessels
- No evidence for inflammation or neoplasia

Clinical Issues
Presentation
- Most common = severely incapacitating postural headache
- Less common
  o Abducens (CN VI) palsy
  o Visual disturbances
- Rare: Severe encephalopathy with disturbed consciousness, death
- LP shows low CSF pressure +/- pleocytosis, increased protein

Natural History
- 75% resolve spontaneously within 3 months (dural thickening, venous engorgement disappear; fluid collections resorbed)
- 20-25% persistent leak, chronic headaches

Treatment
- Conservative Rx to restore CSF volume (fluid replacement, bed rest)
- Other
  o Autologous blood patch
  o Epidural saline infusion
  o Surgery if large dural tear, ruptured diverticulum or Tarlov cyst

Prognosis
- Generally excellent
- Rare: Coma, death from intracranial herniation

Selected References
1. Schrijver I et al: Spontaneous spinal cerebrospinal fluid leaks and minor skeletal features of Marfan syndrome: a microfibrillopathy. J Neurosurg 96: 483-489, 2002
2. Rabin BM et al: Spontaneous intracranial hypotension: Spinal MR findings. AJNR 19: 1034-9, 1998
3. Moayeri NN et al: Spinal dural enhancement on MRI associated with spontaneous intracranial hypotension. J Neurosrug 88: 912-8, 1998

Hardware Follow-up/Failure

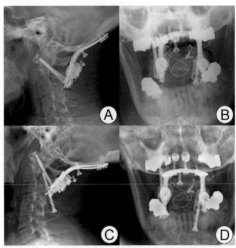

Rheumatoid arthritis. (A, B) Lateral and open-mouth plain films following C0-C2 fusion for C1/2 instability show expected post-operative appearance. (C, D) Follow-up 5 months later for severe neck pain shows that the left transarticular screw has backed out from the left C1 and C2 lateral masses.

Key Facts
- Definition: Malfunction or mechanical breakdown of hardware
- Classic imaging appearance: Broken hardware, or altered location of hardware
- May result in spinal instability
- Important not only to ascertain that hardware has failed but also to look for complicating subluxation or osseous fracture
- Plain films very good for assessing hardware integrity and fusion status
  - Cost effective
  - Abnormalities frequently apparent
  - Abnormal findings can be further evaluated with CT or MRI

Imaging Findings
General Features
- Important to understand expected appearance of properly placed intact hardware
  - References describing normal hardware appearance available
  - Hardware is intended to temporarily stabilize a fusion construct while awaiting successful osseous fusion
  - All hardware will eventually fail if bone fusion does not occur first
- Best imaging clues: Broken or malpositioned hardware, or interval unintended change in spinal alignment
CT Findings
- Best for showing occult fracture and assessing postoperative osseous changes (fusion or hardware loosening)
  - Loosening produces lucency surrounding screws that may be difficult to perceive on plain film but is usually obvious on CT
- Sagittal and coronal reformatted images excellent for assessing alignment and hardware status in complex constructs or osteopenic patients

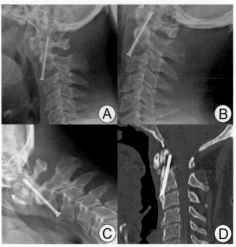

(A) Lateral radiograph following odontoid screw fixation of type II fracture (1 year previously) shows persistent lucency at dens base. Extension (B), flexion (C) views show anterior C1 ring, dens travel independently of C2 base indicating non-union and hardware failure. (D) Sagittal MPR confirms hardware and fusion failure.

MR Findings
- Generally does not show hardware location or integrity well
- Steel hardware produces extensive artifact that makes MR nearly useless
- Modern hardware made of titanium produces minimal artifact
- FSE T1 and T2 techniques minimize artifact
- MRI useful for demonstrating impact on surrounding tissue

Other Modality Findings
- Plain films show spinal alignment and survey hardware integrity
  o Permit cost effective hardware surveillance
- May be done in upright position in dynamic flexion and extension to better simulate hardware integrity during activities of daily living

Imaging Recommendations
- Plain film surveillance
  o Dynamic upright flexion-extension films if hardware failure is questioned
- CT in cases where occult hardware failure is suspected but not clear on plain films
  o Especially helpful with complex constructs and in osteopenic patients
  o Consider sagittal and coronal reformats
- MRI to identify soft-tissue complications or spinal cord injury
  o Avoid GRE or SE sequences; consider FSE technique to minimize artifact

Differential Diagnosis
- None

Pathology
General
- All hardware eventually fails if fusion does not occur in timely fashion

Hardware Follow-up/Failure

- Failure of osseous fusion produces sclerosis and rounding of nonunited fragments
  - Caveat – some patients do form a fibrous union that provides satisfactory stability in absence of radiographic osseous fusion
  - Best confirmed with dynamic plain films
- Fusion rate lower in smokers compared to non-smokers
- Important to consider initial indication for fusion in suspected hardware failure
  - Failed trauma fusion may indicate unsuspected ligamentous injury
  - Failed fusion for neoplasm may indicate tumor progression

Clinical Issues
Presentation
- Frequently asymptomatic; symptomatic presentation usually pain or cord compression

Natural History
- Hardware failure may proceed to fusion even if hardware is broken
- Fibrous union without radiographic solid fusion may be satisfactory
- Best demonstrated with dynamic plain films

Treatment
- Conservative observation or repeat surgical fusion depending on symptoms or clinical findings

Prognosis
- Variable

Selected References
1. Apfelbaum RI et al: Direct anterior screw fixation for recent and remote odontoid fractures. J Neurosurg 93(2 Suppl): 227-36, 2000
2. Lowery GL et al: The significance of hardware failure in anterior cervical plate fixation. Patients with 2- to 7-year follow-up. Spine 23(2): 181-6, discussion 186-7, 1998
3. Slone RM et al: Spinal fixation. Part 3. complications of spinal instrumentation. Radiographics 13(4): 797-816, 1993

Post Surgical Accelerated Degeneration

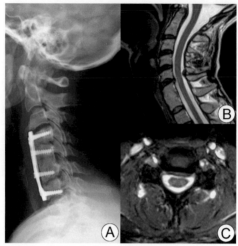

(A) Lateral plain film shows anterior cervical fusion from C4-C7 with accelerated degeneration at C3-4 and C7-T1 levels. (B, C) Sagittal T2WI and axial GRE images show solid C6-7 anterior fusion with C5-6 broad-based herniation and ligamentum flavum redundancy.

Key Facts
- Synonym(s): Spinal "transitional" degenerative syndrome, accelerated segmental degeneration
- Definition: Accelerated degeneration of disc space and facets at level(s) adjacent to surgical fusion
- Classic imaging appearance: Degenerative disc and facet changes directly above or below fusion
  - Also occurs adjacent to congenital segmentation anomalies
- Produced by aberrant biophysical stresses from altered normal spinal motion
  - More common with multilevel fusion, but also seen following single level fusion

Imaging Findings
General Features
- Best imaging clue: Degenerative disc and facet changes directly adjacent to fused vertebra
CT Findings
- Typical findings seen in degenerative disc and facet disease
MR Findings
- Typical findings seen in degenerative disc and facet disease
Other Modality Findings
- Plain films show surgical with adjacent segment degenerative changes
Imaging Recommendations
- Plain films most economical way to demonstrate presence of adjacent segment degenerative changes and to serially follow for progression
- MRI best identifies soft tissue abnormalities that are occult on plain film
  - Disc herniation, ligamentum flavum redundancy, synovial proliferation

Post Surgical Accelerated Degeneration

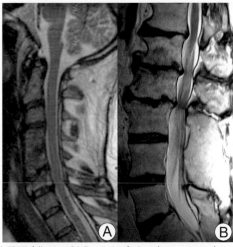

(A) Sagittal T2WI following C4-5 anterior fusion shows severe degenerative disc changes at C5-6. (B) Sagittal T2WI following L3-S1 posterior fusion shows solid fusion mass and severe degenerative changes at T12-L1, L1-2, and L2-3.

Differential Diagnosis
- None

Pathology
General
- General Path Comments
  - Not all patients at risk demonstrate accelerated degeneration
  - Pathological findings are typical of degenerative disc and facet disease
- Etiology-Pathogenesis
  - A solid fusion alters biomechanics at adjacent mobile levels
  - Increased mobility in these remaining mobile segments is hypothesized to cause accelerated degenerative pathologic changes
- Epidemiology
  - More common after surgical fusion than following decompression only

Clinical Issues
Presentation
- Radicular or myelopathic symptoms referable to level(s) above or below a surgical fusion
- Mechanical pain
Natural History
- Progressively worsens
Treatment
- Surgical decompression and fusion at adjacent symptomatic levels
Prognosis
- Variable

Post Surgical Accelerated Degeneration

Selected References
1. Farcy JP: Review of surgical cases which have deteriorated over time. Bull Acad Natl Med 183(4): 775-82, 1999
2. Eck JC et al: Adjacent-segment degeneration after lumbar fusion: a review of clinical, biomechanical, and radiologic studies. Am J Orthop 28(6): 336-40, 1999
3. Wu W et al: Degenerative changes following anterior cervical discectomy and fusion evaluated by fast spin-echo MR imaging. Acta Radiol 37(5): 614-7, 1996

Peridural Fibrosis

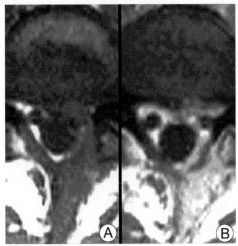

Axial pre- (A) and post-gadolinium (B) T1WI at L4-5 demonstrates enhancing epidural fibrotic tissue ventral to the thecal sac and the traversing left L5 nerve root. The patient is status post laminectomy. Enhancing scar tissue is also present posteriorly.

Key Facts
- Synonym: Epidural fibrosis
- Definition: Scar formation after lumbar surgery
- Classic imaging appearance: Enhancing epidural soft tissue surrounding the typically enlarged nerve root
- 10% rate of recurrent back/radicular pain 6 months after discectomy
  - Failed back syndrome
- Causes of recurrent pain
  - Recurrent disc herniation
  - New herniation at another level
  - Peridural fibrosis
    - Up to one-quarter of all failed back syndrome cases
    - Whether a source of recurrent pain is still controversial
    - Most patients with some degree of fibrosis are asymptomatic
    - One prospective multicenter study (1996) shows that patients with extensive peridural fibrosis are 3.2 times more likely to have recurrent radicular pain than those with less extensive scarring
- An implantable gel (ADCON-L) has been shown to
  - Minimize the formation of peridural fibrotic tissue
  - Decrease the occurrence of pain
    - In two large prospective randomized multicenter trials
  - Acts as a resorbable deterrent to fibroblast ingrowth
- Pre- and post-gadolinium enhanced MRI approximately 96% accurate in differentiating peridural fibrosis from disc herniation

Imaging Findings
General Features
- Best imaging clue

Peridural Fibrosis

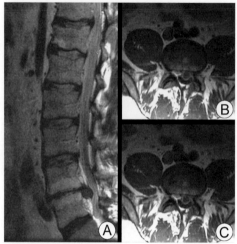

In a second patient, a recurrent disc extrusion (A, B) with peripheral post-gadolinium enhancement (C) is present at L4-5.

- o Infiltration of epidural and perineural fat by soft tissue density (intensity)
- o Can be mass like
- o Immediate homogeneous post-contrast enhancement

CT Findings
- Epidural soft tissue density
  - o Enhances after intravenous contrast

MR Findings
- Peridural soft-tissue intensity
  - o +/- Mass effect
  - o Often surrounds a nerve root
  - o Isointense on T1WI
  - o Variable signal intensity on T2WI
  - o Post-gadolinium enhancement
    - Enhancement regardless the time elapsed since surgery
- Involved nerve root may show post-gadolinium enhancement
- A combination of disc and scar may be present
- Post-surgical changes in the posterior elements

Imaging Recommendations
- Fat suppression of T1WI (pre- and post-gadolinium) may increase sensitivity
  - o In detecting peridural fibrosis and differentiating fibrosis from disc

Differential Diagnosis

Recurrent Disc Herniation
- No central enhancement when imaged early after intravenous gadolinium
  - o Peripheral enhancement common
- Delayed central enhancement if imaged after 30 minutes or later
  - o Diffusion of contrast into disc

Peridural Fibrosis

Pathology

<u>General</u>
- General Path Comments
  - o Postoperative scarring is a part of normal reparative mechanism
- Etiology-Pathogenesis
  - o The extent of fibrosis possibly related to the extent of surgical dissection
  - o The degree of host inflammatory response also plays a role
  - o Scar tissue compresses, irritates, and puts abnormal traction on the nerve roots
    - ▪ Blood supply compromised
    - ▪ Axoplasmic transport interrupted

Clinical Issues

<u>Presentation</u>
- Low back or radicular pain
- Numbness
- Weakness

<u>Treatment</u>
- Periradicular injection of corticosteroids and local anesthetics
- Spinal cord stimulation by implanted electrodes
- Surgical lysis of scar tissue

<u>Prognosis</u>
- 30% to 35% success rate for repeat surgery
- 50% to 70% success rate for spinal cord stimulation

Selected References
1. Ross JS et al: Association between peridural scar and recurrent radicular pain after lumbar discectomy: Magnetic resonance evaluation. Neurosurgery 38: 855-61, 1996
2. Ross JS et al: MR imaging of the postoperative lumbar spine: assessment with gadopentate dimeglumine. AJR 155: 867-72, 1990
3. Hueftle MG et al: Lumbar spine: postoperative MR imaging with Gd-DTPA. Radiology 167: 817-24, 1988

VASCULAR LESIONS

Dural Arteriovenous Fistula

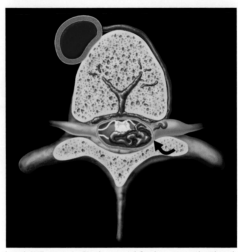

Intradural dorsal AVF, type A. Single arterial feeder enters the thecal sac through the left neural foramen root sleeve and drains through a dilated intradural vein via a single arteriovenous connection (arrow). Note conus compression, myelopathy.

Key Facts
- Synonym(s): DAVF, Dural AVF, Type I AVM
- Definition: Spinal AV fistula, usually dorsal intradural
- Classic imaging appearance: Abnormally enlarged and T2 hyperintense distal cord covered with dilated pial veins
- 80% of spinal vascular malformations
- Typical patient presents in third to sixth decade with progressive lower extremity weakness exacerbated by exercise
- No association with other CNS vascular malformations
- Imaging and clinical findings are frequently subtle or nonspecific; early diagnosis requires a high level of suspicion

Imaging Findings
General Features
- Most commonly occur at level of conus
- Best imaging clue: Small dilated pial veins on the dorsal or ventral surface of a swollen T2 hyperintense distal cord/conus
CT Findings
- Enlarged distal spinal cord
- Enhancing pial veins on cord surface
- Much more difficult to diagnose on CT than MR imaging
MR Findings
- T1WI – cord enlargement and abnormal hypointensity
  - Abnormal small enhancing vessels on cord pial surface
- T2WI – cord enlargement and abnormal hyperintensity
  - Multiple small abnormal vessel flow voids (dilated pial veins) on the cord pial surface
- Occasionally MR imaging is normal or demonstrates abnormal cord signal only

Dural Arteriovenous Fistula

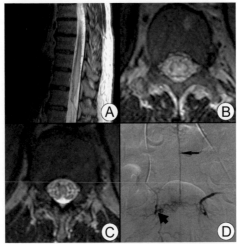

DAVF. Sagittal (A) and axial (B, C) T2WI show enlargement and abnormal T2 hyperintensity of the distal cord and conus representing venous hypertension. Note numerous pial vein flow voids. (D) Selective catheter angiogram reveals AVF (wide arrow) with draining perimedullary vein (arrow).

Other Modality Findings
- Spinal arteriography is gold standard for confirming diagnosis
  - Permits identification of exact level of arteriovenous shunt
  - Provides access for interventional therapy

Imaging Recommendations
- First perform focused MR imaging with small field of view and thin slices in both sagittal (3 mm/0 mm gap) and axial planes (4 mm/0 mm gap)
  - T1WI, T2WI, and enhanced T1WI sequences in both planes
- Use selective spinal arteriography to confirm diagnosis and direct treatment planning

Differential Diagnosis

Spinal Cord Arteriovenous Malformation (SCAVM)
- Usually acute presentation (compared to insidious presentation of DAVF)
- Intramedullary or subarachnoid hemorrhage relatively common

Amyotrophic Lateral Sclerosis
- Usually distinguished from DAVF by eliciting specific clinical features
- Brain MR imaging may be characteristically abnormal

Cervical or Thoracic Spondylosis/Disc Disease
- Distinguishable clinically and by imaging

Pathology

General
- General Path Comments
  - Lesions are extramedullary AVFs, not true AVMs
    - No intervening small vessel network
    - Fistula drains directly into venous outflow tract
    - Usually intradural
  - Supplied by small tortuous arteries originating from the dura mater

Dural Arteriovenous Fistula

- Etiology-Pathogenesis
  - Postulated to be acquired lesions, possibly from thrombosis of extradural venous system
  - Venous drainage from the DAVF results in increased pial vein pressure that is transmitted to the intrinsic cord veins
  - Venous hypertension from engorgement reduces intramedullary AV pressure gradient, causing reduced tissue perfusion and cord ischemia
- Epidemiology
  - 80% of patients are male
  - Usually presents in 4th or 5th decade
    - Range: Ages 20s through 80s

Gross Pathologic-Surgical Features
- Most commonly occurs at the thoracolumbar level (T5-L3)
- Usually located either adjacent to the intervertebral foramen or within the dural root sleeve
- Arterial supply arises from dural branch of a radicular artery
- Intradural vein drains directly into the cord pial veins
- Frequently poor correlation between the location of the AV shunt and the clinical level of spinal dysfunction
- Rarely, clinically manifests as "subacute necrotizing myelopathy" ("Foux-Alajounine syndrome")

Staging or Grading Criteria
- Previously categorized as Type IV spinal arteriovenous malformation
  - Misnomer that implies a true AVM etiology rather than AVF

Clinical Issues

Presentation
- Most common presentation is progressive lower extremity weakness with both upper and lower motor neuron involvement
- Additional symptoms include back pain, bowel/bladder dysfunction, and impotence
- Thoracolumbar fistula location spares upper extremities
- Never presents with hemorrhage

Natural History
- Slowly progressive clinical course over several years leading to paraplegia

Treatment
- Endovascular fistula occlusion with permanent embolic agents
- Surgical fistula obliteration

Prognosis
- Cord ischemia is reversible if treated early, but may become irreversible when untreated
- Bowel/bladder dysfunction and impotence rarely improve, even after successful obliteration of fistula

Selected References
1. Spetzler RF et al: Modified classification of spinal cord vascular lesions. J Neurosurg (Spine 2) 96: 145-156, 2002
2. Connors J et al: Interventional Neuroradiology. 1st ed. Philadelphia: W.B. Saunders, 1999
3. Anson J et al: Classification of spinal arteriovenous malformations and implications for treatment. BNI Quarterly 8: 2-8, 1992

Arteriovenous Malformation

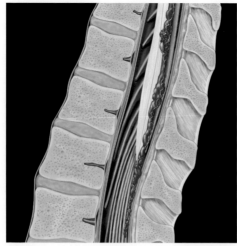

Sagittal graphic depicts a subpial juvenile (type III) cord AVM. Note "scalloped" appearance of the dorsal cord caused by enlarged draining veins. Chronic venous hypertension has caused cord atrophy.

Key Facts

- Definition: Direct arterial/venous communications without capillary bed
- Traditional classification
  - Type I: Dural arteriovenous fistula (DAVF)(see DAVF Dx)
  - Type II: Intramedullary glomus type AVM (similar to brain AVM)
  - Type III: Juvenile-type AVM (intramedullary, extramedullary)
  - Type IV: Intradural extra/perimedullary AVF (Types A, B, C)
- Newest classification of AVMs into extra-intradural; intradural (intramedullary, compact, diffuse, conus; subtyped by flow, size)
- AVMs account for < 10% of spinal masses
  - Most common = Type I (up to 80%)
  - Second most common = Intramedullary, Type II, III (15-20%)
- Imaging: Prominent "flow voids" + variable cord atrophy/gliosis

Imaging Findings

General Features

- Best imaging clue: Flow voids with cord hyperintensity (Type I)
  - Type II: Intramedullary nidus (may extend to dorsal subpial surface)
  - Type III: Nidus may have extramedullary and extraspinal extension
  - Type IV: Ventral fistula (venous varices displace, distort cord)

CT Findings

- NECT: Usually normal (rare = widened interpedicular distance, posterior vertebral scalloping)
- CECT: May show enlarged cord with enhancing nidus, pial vessels (rare)

MR Findings

- Types II, III (intramedullary AVMs)
  - T1WI: Large cord, heterogeneous signal (blood products), flow voids
  - T2WI: Cord hyperintense (edema, gliosis, ischemia) or mixed (blood)
  - Contrast enhanced T1WI: Variable enhancement of nidus, cord, vessels
- Type IV (perimedullary)

Arteriovenous Malformation

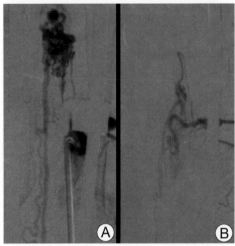

A 22-year-old female with scoliosis and progressive myelopathy after fixation. Spinal angiography demonstrates a compact vascular nidus supplied mostly by left T9 (A) radicular artery. Some supply comes from T8 (B). Type II (glomus) AVM.

- o T1WI: Ventral fistula, large flow voids distort/displace cord
- o T2WI: Hyperintense cord + flow voids
- o Contrast: Enhancing pial vessels, epidural plexus, +/- patchy enhancement distal cord

Other Modality Findings
- DSA
  - o Type II: Supplied by anterior spinal artery (ASA) or posterior spinal artery (PSA); nidus drains to coronal venous plexus (on cord surface) which in turn drains anterograde to extradural space
  - o Type III: Large complex nidus, multiple feeding vessels; may be intramedullary and extramedullary and even extraspinal
  - o Type IV: Feeding vessel from ASA or PSA connects directly with spinal vein (no nidus!)
- Myelography (intramedullary/perimedullary AVMs): Serpentine filling defects along posterior cord

Imaging Recommendations
- Contrast-enhanced MRI; consider spinal angiography +/- embolization

Differential Diagnosis
Intramedullary Neoplasm
- Ependymoma: Heterogeneous (cysts, blood products)
- Astrocytoma: Multisegmental enhancing mass, no enlarged vessels

Pathology
General
- General Path Comments
  - o Location
    - ▪ Type II (glomus): Cervical/upper thoracic (may occur anywhere)
    - ▪ Type III (juvenile): Cervical/upper thoracic (may occur anywhere)

Arteriovenous Malformation

- Type IV: Conus medullaris (type A,B), thoracic (type C)
- Genetics (can be sporadic or syndromic)
  - Type II: Associated with cutaneous angiomas, Klippel-Trenaunay-Weber, Rendu-Osler-Weber syndromes
  - Type III: Associated with Cobb's syndrome (metameric vascular malformation involving triad of spinal cord, skin, bone)
  - Type IV: Associated with Rendu-Osler-Weber syndrome
- Embryology
  - Persistence of primitive direct communications between arterial and venous channels, without intervening capillary bed
- Etiology-Pathogenesis
  - Type II: Compact nidus, high-flow, aneurysms common (20-44%)
  - Type III: Large diffuse nidus, cord ischemia, venous hypertension
  - Type IV: Congenital; may be acquired after trauma; (A) venous hypertension, (B,C) arterial steal, (C) cord compression
- Epidemiology
  - Intramedullary (Type II, III):15-20% of spinal AVM; Type IV:10-20%

Gross Pathologic-Surgical Features

- Type II: Compact intramedullary nidus lacks normal capillary bed; no parenchyma within nidus; (nidus may have pial extension)
- Type III: Large, complex intramedullary lesion, normal neural parenchyma inside nidus (may involve extramedullary, extradural)
- Type IV: Direct fistula between ASA/PSA & draining vein, no nidus
  - IV-A: Small AVF with slow flow, mild venous enlargement
  - IV-B: Intermediate AVF, dilated feeding arteries; high flow rate
  - IV-C: Large AVF, dilated feeding arteries; dilated, tortuous veins

Microscopic Features

- Abnormal vessels with variable wall thickness, internal elastic lamina
- Reactive change in surrounding tissue: gliosis, cytoid bodies, Rosenthal fibers; hemosiderin deposition common; +/- Ca++

Clinical Issues

Presentation

- Type II: M=F, 20-40y, SAH most common symptom; pain, myelopathy
- Type III: M=F, < 30y, progressive neurologic decline (weakness), SAH
- Type IV: M=F, 10-40y, progressive conus /cauda equina syndrome, SAH

Treatment

- Type II: Surgical resection, + pre-op embolization (aneurysms, nidus)
- Type III: Complete resection generally not possible, palliative therapy
- Type IV: Embolization or surgical resection: (A) surgical resection, (B) surgical resection or embolization, (C) embolization

Prognosis

- Good outcome in Type II (glomus) and IV (perimedullary)
- Poor prognosis for juvenile (Type III) AVM

Selected References
1.   Spetzler RF et al: Modified classification of spinal cord vascular lesions. J Neurosurg (Spine 2) 96: 145-156, 2002
2.   Bemporad JA et al: Magnetic resonance imaging of spinal cord vascular malformations with an emphasis on the cervical spine. In Neuropathic basis for imaging. Neuroimaging Clinics of North America 11:111-29, 2001
3.   Bao YH et al: Classification and therapeutic modalities of spinal vascular malformations in 80 patients. Neurosurgery 40:75-81, 1997

Cavernous Malformation

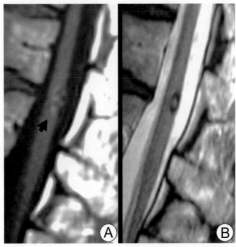

A 40-year-old female with progressive myelopathy. (A) Sagittal T1WI shows a small focal mass with "popcorn" appearance (arrow) caused by blood products of varying ages. (B) T2WI shows a dark hemosiderin rim, typical for a cavernous malformation.

Key Facts
- Synonym(s): Cavernous angioma
- Definition: Vascular lesion with lobulated, thin sinusoidal vascular channels, no interspersed neural tissue
- Spinal cord uncommon site, 3-5% of all cavernous malformations (CMs)
- Imaging: Heterogeneous mass ("locules" of blood with "popcorn" appearance) surrounded by dark rim (hemosiderin)
- Familial CMs at high risk for hemorrhage, forming new lesions

Imaging Findings
General Features
- Best imaging clue: Locules of blood with fluid-fluid levels surrounded by very hypointense rim
- Extremely rare: Subarachnoid hemorrhage
CT Findings
- NECT: Often normal; cord may appear widened
- CECT: +/- faint enhancement (rare)
MR Findings
- T1WI: Heterogeneous (blood products, varying ages)
- T2WI: Heterogeneous, hypointense rim (hemosiderin)
- Gradient-echo (GRE): Prominent "blooming"
- Contrast enhanced T1WI: Enhancement absent/minimal
Other Modality Findings
- DSA: Negative (one of "angiographically occult" vascular malformations)
Imaging Recommendations
- MRI spine (use GRE, contrast sequences to exclude other etiologies)
- Scan the brain (may show other lesions)!

Cavernous Malformation

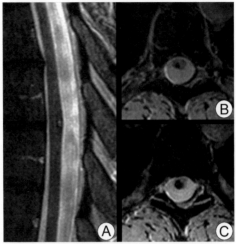

A 50-year-old female with sensorimotor deficits. Sagittal and axial T2WI (A, B) show the heterogeneous lesion in the posterior cord with a dark hemosiderin rim. (C) Axial GRE image shows typical signal "blooming."

Differential Diagnosis
Intramedullary Neoplasm
- Ependymoma: Enhancing mass with cysts, blood products
- Astrocytoma: Multisegmental enhancing mass (hemorrhage uncommon)
- Hemangioblastoma: Vascular nodule; "flow voids" common
AVM
- Enlarged flow voids with vascular nidus
- DSA reveals enlarged feeding arteries, nidus, early draining veins

Pathology
General
- General Path Comments
  - Identical to intracranial cavernous malformations
  - Location: Thoracic > cervical > lumbar
- Genetics
  - Multiple (familial) CM syndrome (50%)
    - Autosomal dominant, variable penetrance
    - Mutation in chromosomes 3, 7q
- Etiology-Pathogenesis
  - Angiogenically immature lesions with endothelial proliferation, increased neoangiogenesis; VEGF, βFGF, TGFα expressed
- Epidemiology
  - 10-30% multiple, familial
  - 70% of spinal CMs in females
Gross Pathologic-Surgical Features
- Discrete, lobulated blue-reddish brown ("mulberry-like") nodule
- Pseudocapsule (gliotic, hemosiderin-stained cord)
Microscopic Features
- Thin-walled epithelial–lined spaces embedded in collagenous matrix

Cavernous Malformation

- Blood products in different stages of evolution
- Ca++ rare (common in brain CMs)

Clinical Issues
<u>Presentation</u>
- Between 3rd and 6th decade
  - Range = 12-88y
  - Peak = 4th decade
- F:M = 2:1
- Most common symptom = sensorimotor deficits, progressive paraparesis
- Four clinical patterns
  - Multiple episodes of neurological deterioration, intermittent recovery
  - Slowly progressive neurological decline
  - Sudden symptom onset with rapid decline (hours-days)
  - Mild symptoms with acute onset, gradual decline (weeks-months)

<u>Natural History</u>
- Broad range of dynamic behavior (may progress, enlarge, regress)
- **De novo** lesions may develop (especially in familial CM syndrome)
- Clinical course varies from slow progression to acute quadriplegia

<u>Treatment</u>
- Surgical resection
- Conservative management if asymptomatic (follow with serial MRIs)

<u>Prognosis</u>
- Postoperative outcome related to preoperative neurologic status
- 66% improved, 28% stable, 6% deterioration postoperatively

Selected References
1. Clatterbuck RE et al: The nature and fate of punctate (Type IV) cavernous malformations. Neurosurg 49:26-32, 2001
2. Sure U et al: Endothelial proliferation, neoangiogenesis, and potential de novo generation of cerebrovascular malformations. J Neurosurg 94:972-7, 2001
3. Zevgaridis D et al: Cavernous hemangiomas of the spinal cord. A review of 117 cases. Acta Neurochir (Wein) 141:237-45, 1999

Spontaneous Epidural Hematoma

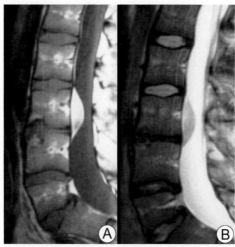

Sagittal T1- (A) and T2WI (B) in a patient with subacute spinal epidural hematoma (EDH). Note the broad-based lentiform configuration and moderate canal stenosis. The EDH is probably venous rather than arterial (case courtesy C. Looney).

Key Facts
- Definition: Epidural hemorrhage (EDH) without apparent cause
- Classic imaging appearance: Loculated spindle-shaped expansion of epidural space with hyperdense appearance on CT, age-dependent altered intensity on MRI
- Other key facts
  - Cervical, thoracic, or lumbar spinal involvement
  - Ventral or dorsal to the thecal sac
  - Variable cranial-caudal dimension
  - MRI should be the initial imaging modality
  - Spinal angiography not indicated unless findings of arteriovenous malformation are present on MRI
  - Early diagnosis and prompt treatment improve prognosis

Imaging Findings
General Features
- Best imaging clue: Extradural multisegmental fluid collection with signal characteristic of blood on MRI, without focal mass, bone lesion, flow voids, or cord tumor

MR Findings
- Epidural mass
  - Acute (< 48 hrs) EDH more commonly iso- than hyperintense to cord on TIWI
  - Subacute and chronic EDH usually hyper- rather than isointense on T1WI
  - Heterogeneously hyperintense on T2WI with central hypointense foci possibly due to deoxyhemoglobin or fibrous septae in the spinal canal
- Peripheral, and occasionally central enhancement after intravenous gadolinium

Spontaneous Epidural Hematoma

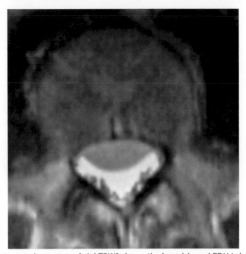

Same case as previous page. Axial T2WI shows the broad-based EDH is hypointense compared to CSF. Moderate compression of the thecal sac is present. No bony erosion or other lesions are identified. Spontaneous EDH.

- o Peripheral enhancement possibly related to adjacent dural hyperemia
- o Central enhancement may be due to leaky vessel with contrast extravasation or enhancing epidural septa
- Mass effect on the cord with cord edema rarely present

Differential Diagnosis
Epidural Abscess
- Associated with infectious spondylitis
- Diffuse enhancement in phlegmon and peripheral enhancement in abscess
Epidural Metastasis
- Diffuse enhancement
- More focal
- Adjacent osseous involvement
- Lymphoma usually not as hyperintense on T2WI due to high nuclear to cytoplasmic ratio
Disc Extrusion, Migration
- Parent disc typically protruding
- Less vertical extent
- Occasionally, EDH associated with disc extrusion, inseparable on imaging

Pathology
General
- Etiology-Pathogenesis
  - o Minor trauma
    - ▪ With possible rupture of the epidural venous plexus
  - o Anticoagulation or coagulopathy
  - o Transient venous hypertension (sudden Valsalva, etc)
  - o Disk herniation
  - o Arteriovenous malformation

Spontaneous Epidural Hematoma

- Epidemiology
  - o Incidence of approximately 0.1 patient per 100,000 patients per year
  - o Less than 1% of the spinal space-occupying lesions
  - o Male predominance
  - o Fifth decade of life or older

Gross Pathologic-Surgical Features
- Isolated epidural hematoma

Clinical Issues

Presentation
- Acute onset of severe pain, radiculopathy
- Progressive paraplegia
- Sensory deficit
- Cauda equina syndrome

Natural History
- May resolve spontaneously

Treatment
- Decompressive laminectomy with clot evacuation
- Nonoperative management
  - o In cases of mild symptoms at presentation, regardless of the degree of cord compression on MRI

Prognosis
- Severity and duration of the neurologic deficits predictive of the degree of neurologic recovery
- Favorable clinical and imaging outcome with conservative management

Selected References
1. Fukui MB et al: Acute spontaneous spinal epidural hematoma. AJNR 20:1365-1372, 1999
2. Alexiadou-Rudolf C et al: Acute nontraumatic spinal epidural hematomas: An important differential diagnosis in spinal emergencies. Spine 23:1810-1813, 1998
3. Holtas S et al: Spontaneous spinal epidural hematoma: Findings at MR imaging and clinical correlation. Radiology 199:409-413, 1996

Spinal Subdural Hematoma

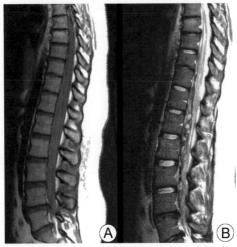

Sagittal T1WI (A) and T2WI (B) demonstrate an anterior intraspinal collection extending from T11 to L4, exerting mass effect on the cauda equina. It is isointense on T1, heterogeneous (iso- and hypointense) on T2.

Key Facts
- Definition: Hemorrhage into the spinal subdural space
- Classic imaging appearance: Lobulated intradural collection predominately hypointense on T2WI or gradient-echo imaging, hyperdense on CT
- Other key facts
  - Less common than epidural hematoma
  - Other than trauma, lumbar puncture in patients with coagulopathy is the most common cause
  - Most common in the lumbar or thoracolumbar spine, with variable cranial-caudal extension
  - Early diagnosis and prompt treatment improve prognosis

Imaging Findings

General Features
- Best imaging clue: Collection bounded by the dura, with a large portion being hypointense on T2WI or gradient-echo imaging

CT Findings
- Hyperdense intradural collection
- Spine fractures in trauma patients

MR Findings
- Variable signal intensity on T1WI and T2WI, from hypo- to iso- to hyperintense
- Significant portion demonstrates hypointensity on T2WI or gradient-echo imaging
- No postgadolinium enhancement
- Variable mass effect on the spinal cord and the cauda equina
- Spinal cord injury usually hyperintense on T2WI with hypointensity suggesting hemorrhagic contusion
- Posttraumatic disc herniation

Spinal Subdural Hematoma

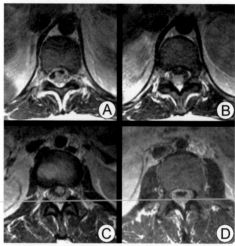

Axial T2WI (A to D) confirm the subdural location and the mass effect on the cauda equina.

Differential Diagnosis

<u>Epidural Hematoma</u>

- "Capping" of the hematoma by the surrounding epidural fat on sagittal imaging
- Obtuse angle between the cerebral spinal fluid within the thecal sac and the hematoma on sagittal imaging
- Directly adjacent to the osseous structures with effacement of the epidural fat

<u>CNS Drop Metastases</u>

- Hyperintense on T2WI
- Postgadolinium enhancement, diffuse and sheet-like, or focal and nodular

Pathology

<u>General</u>

- Embryology-Anatomy
  - Inner dural layer is structurally weaker than the outer layer
    - May tear open during trauma, accommodating "subdural" hemorrhage
  - True spinal subdural space has been demonstrated in human autopsy studies
- Etiology-Pathogenesis
  - Trauma
  - Anticoagulation or coagulopathy
  - Iatrogenic causes, especially in the presence of abnormal coagulation parameters
    - Lumbar puncture
    - Spinal anesthesia
  - Neoplasm
  - Arteriovenous malformation
  - Idiopathic

Spinal Subdural Hematoma

- Epidemiology
  - M:F = 1:1
  - Fifth decade or older

Clinical Issues

Presentation
- Acute onset of severe back pain
- Neurologic impairment may be delayed
  - Radiculopathy
  - Paraplegia
  - Sensory deficits
  - Sphincter dysfunction

Natural History
- May resolve spontaneously

Treatment
- Decompressive laminectomy with clot evacuation
- Nonoperative management in cases of mild symptoms at presentation

Prognosis
- Over forty percent of the patients undergoing surgery will have favorable outcome
- Concurrent subarachnoid hemorrhage portends poor outcome
- Favorable clinical and imaging result with conservative management

Selected References
1. Domenicucci M et al: Nontraumatic acute spinal subdural hematoma: Report of five cases and review of the literature. J Neurosurg 91:65-73, 1999
2. Longatti PL et al: Spontaneous spinal subdural hematoma. Journal of Neurosurgical Sciences 38:197-9, 1994
3. Donovan MJ et al: Acute spinal subdural hematoma: MR and CT findings with pathologic correlates. AJNR 15:1895-905, 1994

Spinal Cord Infarction

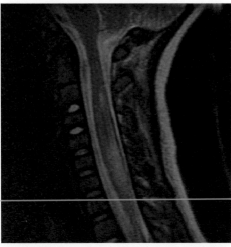

Sagittal T2WI in a child with spinal cord infarct shows expansion, hyperintensity of the cervical cord extending from C3 to C7.

Key Facts
- Definition: Permanent tissue loss in the spinal cord due to vessel occlusion, typically a radicular branch of the vertebral artery (cervical cord) or the aorta (thoracic and lumbar cord)
- Classic imaging appearance: T2 hyperintensity involving the anterior horn cells
- Other key facts
  - Most frequent in the upper thoracic cord because of arterial border zone
  - Sudden onset of neurologic deficits helps to make the diagnosis
  - Anterior spinal syndrome presents with paralysis, loss of pain and temperature sensation, and bladder and bowel dysfunction
  - Posterior spinal cord infarction characterized by loss of proprioception and vibration sense, paresis, and sphincter dysfunction
  - Anterior sulcus artery occlusion presents with Brown-Sequard syndrome

Imaging Findings
<u>General Features</u>
- Best imaging clue: Focal hyperintensity on T2WI in slightly expanded cord
<u>MR Findings</u>
- Normal or slightly expansile spinal cord
- Atrophy in late stage
- No significant T1 signal abnormality
- T2 hyperintensity in the gray matter, the gray matter with adjacent white matter, or the entire cross sectional area of the cord
- Focal hemorrhage conversion may occur with hyperintensity on T1WI and hypointensity on T2WI
- Mild focal and patchy post-gadolinium enhancement in subacute phase

Spinal Cord Infarction

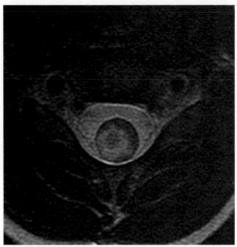

Same case as previous page. Axial T2WI shows cord expansion, hyperintensity. Only a small part of the peripheral cord is spared, probably with flow from small radicular collateral vessels. The slightly more hypointense center may represent hemorrhage (case courtesy G. Hedlund).

- May see large vessel abnormalities such as aortic aneurysm or dissection
- Marrow T2 hyperintensity in the anterior vertebral body or in the deep medullary portion near the endplate may be present due to vertebral body infarct

Other Modality Findings
- Spinal artery occlusion on angiography
- Dissection or aneurysm in appropriate artery on MRA or catheter angiography

Differential Diagnosis
Multiple Sclerosis
- Peripheral in location
- Less than two vertebral segments in length
- Less than half the cross-sectional area of the cord
- 90% incidence of associated intracranial lesions
- Relapsing and remitting clinical course

Spinal Cord Neoplasm
- Cord expansion invariably present
- Diffuse or nodular contrast enhancement
- Extensive peri-tumoral edema
- Associated cystic changes
- Slower clinical onset

Idiopathic Transverse Myelitis
- Lesion centrally located
- 3 to 4 segments in length
- Occupying more than two thirds of the cord's cross-sectional area
- No associated intracranial lesions
- Onset not quite as sudden

Spinal Cord Infarction

Pathology

General

- Embryology-Anatomy
  - Seven to eight of the 62 (31 pairs) radicular arteries supply the spinal cord in three territories
  - Cervicothoracic territory includes the cervical cord and the first two or three thoracic segments, supplied by anterior spinal artery from the vertebral artery and branches of the costocervical trunk
  - Midthoracic territory includes the fourth to eighth thoracic segments, supplied by a radicular branch from the aorta at the T7 level
  - Thoracolumbar territory includes the remainder of the thoracic segments and the lumbar cord, supplied by the artery of Adamkiewicz
  - The artery of Adamkiewicz usually originates from the 9th, 10th, 11th, or 12th intercostal artery (75%), less commonly from the higher intercostal artery or a lumbar artery
  - The radicular arteries form one anterior and two posterior spinal arteries
  - The anterior spinal arteries and branches supply the gray matter and an adjacent mantle of white matter
  - The posterior spinal arteries and branches supply one third to one half of the periphery of the cord
- Etiology-Pathogenesis
  - Idiopathic
  - Atherosclerosis
  - Thoracoabdominal aneurysm
  - Aortic surgery
  - Systemic hypotension
  - Infection
  - Embolic disease
  - Spinal arteriovenous malformation
- Epidemiology
  - Rare, usually patients > 50

Clinical Issues

Presentation

- Abrupt onset of weakness and loss of sensation
- Rapid progression of neurologic deficits, reaching maximum impairment within hours

Treatment

- Anticoagulation
- Intravenous corticosteroids
- Maintain systemic perfusion
- Physical rehabilitation

Prognosis

- Poor with limited recovery of neurologic function

Selected References
1. Yuh WT et al: MR imaging of spinal cord and vertebral body infarction. AJNR 13:145-154, 1992
2. Berlit P et al: Spinal cord infarction: MRI and MEP findings in three cases. Journal of Spinal Disorders 5:212-216, 1992
3. Mawad ME et al: Spinal cord ischemia after resection of thoracoabdominal aortic aneurysms: MR findings in 24 patients. AJNR 11:987-991, 1990

VERTEBRAL MARROW CHANGES

Hyperplastic Vertebral Marrow

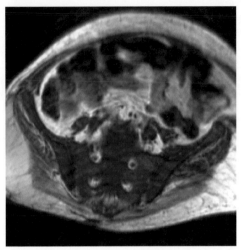

Axial T1WI of the sacrum and iliac wings in a patient with chronic anemia, fever, high white count, and high erythrocyte sedimentation rate demonstrates diffuse hypointense marrow signal intensity, lower than the surrounding muscles.

Key Facts
- Synonyms: Expanded marrow; Marrow reconversion
- Definition: Reconversion of fatty marrow to red marrow in the presence of chronic anemia
- Classic imaging appearance: Diffuse hypointense marrow on T1WI
- Process of reconversion starts in the axial skeleton
  - Beginning with skull, then vertebrae, ribs, sternum, and pelvis
  - Followed by the extremities
    - From proximal to distal
    - Extensive reconversion in the appendicular skeleton suggestive of severe anemia or neoplastic involvement of the axial skeleton

Imaging Findings
General Features
- Best imaging clue: Intervertebral discs hyperintense to vertebral marrow on T1WI
MR Findings
- T1WI: Diffuse or focal diminished signal intensity (SI)
  - Where fatty marrow is expected
  - Similar to muscle SI
  - Normal vertebral marrow SI higher than muscle SI
- T2WI: Variable
  - SI similar to, but not higher than, muscle SI on fat saturated T2WI or STIR
- No post-gadolinium enhancement
Nuclear Medicine Findings
- Tc-99m diphosphonate or Tc-99m sulfur colloid scan
- Sites of increased uptake due to marrow expansion
  - Distal appendicular skeleton
  - Calvarium

Hyperplastic Vertebral Marrow

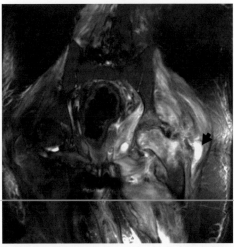

Coronal T2WI with fat saturation in the same patient shows diffuse hypointense marrow. Marrow edema is present in the proximal left femur with surrounding muscle hyperintensities and fluid collections (arrow) due to osteomyelitis, abscesses, and myositis.

Imaging Recommendations
- STIR or T2WI with fat saturation to distinguish hematopoietic elements from marrow edema or neoplastic infiltration
- Pre- and postgadolinium T1WI with fat saturation also helpful

Differential Diagnosis
Marrow Infiltration
- Leukemia, lymphoma, multiple myeloma, or metastases
- Diffuse or focal T1 hypointensity
- SI usually great than muscle SI on STIR or fat suppressed T2WI
- Postgadolinium enhancement
COPD, Obesity (Pickwickian syndrome), or High Altitude
- Marrow SI may be hypointense on T1WI
  - Overlapping with hyperplastic marrow pattern
- Probably due to chronic hypoxemia with increased erythroid production

Pathology
General
- General Path Comments
  - Demand of hematopoiesis exceeds the available cellular marrow
    - Recruitment of yellow marrow to produce red marrow results in the imaging appearance
- Embryology-Anatomy
  - At birth, the marrow space in the entire skeleton is occupied with red marrow
  - Conversion of red to yellow marrow occurs in the next two decades of life
    - From peripheral and distal to central and proximal

- o Adult marrow pattern: Red marrow predominantly in
  - Axial skeleton, proximal humeri, and proximal femora
- o With age, volume of red marrow decreases
  - From 58% of the total marrow volume in the first decade to 29% by the eighth decade
- o The amount of fatty marrow increases
  - Also to replace bone loss
- Etiology-Pathogenesis
  - o Anemia of chronic disease
    - Infections (e.g. AIDS), inflammatory disease (e.g. RA), and cancer most common
    - Interferons and interleukins from monocytes inhibit erythropoietin production and erythroid proliferation
    - Inadequate release of iron from reticulum cells to the plasma
    - Increased destruction of red blood cells by the reticuloendothelial system
  - o Iron deficiency anemia
    - Chronic blood loss
    - Increased requirements (pregnancy, adolescence, etc.)
    - Poor diet
  - o Hemolytic anemia
    - Sickle cell disease
    - Thalassemia
- Epidemiology
  - o Iron deficiency anemia is the most common cause of anemia
  - o Anemia of chronic disease second most common

Microscopic Features
- Anemia of chronic disease
  - o Normal or increased reticuloendothelial iron storage
    - Increased stainable marrow iron in more than 50% of patients with AIDS
- Iron deficiency anemia
  - o Decreased reticuloendothelial iron storage

Clinical Issues
Presentation
- Findings of underlying infectious, inflammatory, or neoplastic process
- Skin and mucous membrane pallor
- Weakness and fatigue
- Dyspnea
- Congestive heart failure

Treatment
- Treatment of the underlying disease causing anemia
- Transfusions
- Recombinant erythropoietin

Prognosis
- Dependent on the underlying etiology causing marrow expansion

Selected References
1. Steiner RM et al: Magnetic resonance imaging of diffuse bone marrow disease. Radiol Clin of North Am 31:383-409, 1993
2. Geremia GK et al: The magnetic resonance hypointense spine of AIDS. J Comput Assist Tomogr 14:785-9, 1990
3. Vogler III JB et al: Bone marrow imaging. Radiology 168:679-93, 1988

Extramedullary Hematopoiesis

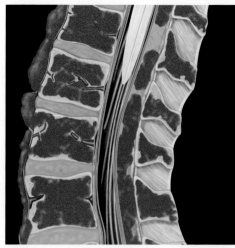

Sagittal illustration of the lumbar spine shows hematopoietic tissue replacing the vertebral marrow and extending into the pre-vertebral and posterior epidural space.

Key Facts

- Definition: Appearance and proliferation of hematopoietic tissue in response to profound chronic anemia, in atypical sites
- Classic imaging appearance
  - Minimally enhancing isointense multi-segmental paraspinal and epidural mass
  - Diffuse marrow hypointensity
- Other key facts
  - Occurs in chronic anemic states
    - Beta-thalassemia (most common)
    - Sickle cell anemia
    - Polycythemia vera
    - Myelofibrosis
    - Myelodysplasia
  - Usually involves the liver, spleen, and kidneys
    - Sites of fetal hematopoiesis
  - May occur in the posterior mediastinum or retroperitoneum
  - Rare in the spine, but when present
    - Thoracic epidural space more commonly involved

Imaging Findings

General Features
- Best imaging clue: Diffuse marrow hypointensity on all sequences

CT Findings
- Nonspecific paraspinal and/or epidural soft-tissue mass narrowing the canal
- Small infarcted spleen in patients with sickle cell disease
- Splenomegaly in other causes

MR Findings
- (Multi-) segmental epidural and/or paravertebral mass

Extramedullary Hematopoiesis

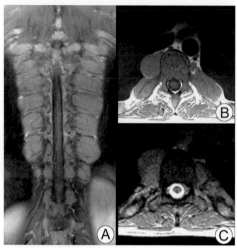

Coronal postgadolinium T1WI with fat saturation of the thoracic spine (A) in a 17 year-old patient with thalassemia demonstrates bilateral paraspinal masses with minimal enhancement. The masses are isointense to muscle on axial T1WI (B) and slightly hyperintense on gradient-echo imaging (C).

- o Iso- to hypointense on T1WI
- o Iso- to hyperintense on T2WI
  - ▪ Hypointensity may represent increased iron content in the hematopoietic tissue
- o Minimal to mild postgadolinium enhancement
- o Variable mass effect on the spinal cord
- Intramedullary T2 hyperintensity may represent edema or myelomalacia

Differential Diagnosis
Epidural/Paraspinal Metastasis
- Contiguous lesion involving the adjacent vertebral body
- Expansion of the involved vertebral body
- Sparing of the spinal column in some cases
- Diffuse vigorous enhancement

Epidural Hematoma
- Isointense to hypointense on T2WI
- Often hyperintense on T1WI
- No post-gadolinium enhancement

Epidural/Paravertebral Abscess
- Associated with infectious spondylitis
- Diffuse or peripheral enhancement

Pathology
General
- Etiology-Pathogenesis
  - o Embryonic hematopoietic rests in the epidural space stimulated in response to chronic severe anemia, versus

Extramedullary Hematopoiesis

- o Direct extension of hematopoietic marrow from the vertebrae into the epidural space

<u>Microscopic Features</u>
- Resembles bone marrow on biopsy
- Erythroid and granulocytic precursors
- Megakaryocytes

Clinical Issues

<u>Presentation</u>
- Symptoms related to chronic anemia
- Chronic back pain
- Paraparesis
- Sensory deficit
- Gait disturbance

<u>Treatment</u>
- Radiation therapy
- Transfusions
- Decompressive laminectomy with surgical resection when neurologically impaired

<u>Prognosis</u>
- Excellent
- Regression of mass with radiation therapy or transfusions

Selected References
1. Dibbern DA et al: MR of thoracic cord compression caused by epidural extramedullary hematopoiesis in myelodysplastic syndrome. AJNR 18:363-6, 1997
2. Kalina P et al: MR of extramedullary hematopoiesis causing cord compression in beta-thalassemia. AJR 13:1408-9, 1992

Multiple Myeloma

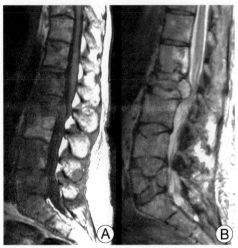

Multiple myeloma. Sagittal T1WI (A) and T2WI (B) of the lumbar spine demonstrate multifocal patchy marrow involvement. Compression deformities involve L2 and L5 vertebral bodies with epidural extension at L2, narrowing the spinal canal.

Key Facts
- Definition: Malignant proliferation of plasma cells in the bone marrow
- Classic imaging appearance: Diffuse osteoperia or multiple punched out lesions on plain film
- Other key facts
  - Most common primary tumor of bone
  - Accounts for 27% of biopsied bone tumors
  - Involvement of bones that contain red marrow: Axial skeleton (spine, skull (mandible), ribs, pelvis) > long bones
  - MRI more sensitive than plain films or bone scintigraphy in assessing disease extent
  - Bone scintigraphy is normal in a majority of cases, detecting 10% of the lesions
  - Plasmocytoma represents early stage of multiple myeloma
    - Presenting in one third of patients, most of them eventually develop multifocal disease, usually within five years
  - POEMS syndrome: Polyneuropathy, organomegaly, endocrine disorders, monoclonal gammopathy, skin changes

Imaging Findings
<u>General Features</u>
- Best imaging clue: Focal, diffuse, or mottled T1 hypointensity
<u>MR Findings</u>
- Normal
- Focal marrow involvement
  - Low to intermediate signal intensity compared to surrounding marrow on T1WI
  - Hyperintense on T2WI or STIR
  - Post-gadolinium enhancement
- Diffuse marrow involvement

Multiple Myeloma

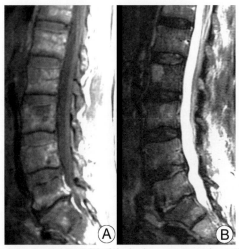

Multiple myeloma. Sagittal T1WI (A) of the lumbar spine in another patient reveals a multifocal patchy marrow pattern. Discrete lesions are better seen on the sagittal STIR image (B).

- o Fatty marrow replaced by low signal intensity, iso- or hypointense to intervertebral discs
- o Diffuse marrow enhancement after intravenous gadolinium
- Variegated pattern
  - o Patchy, heterogeneous, and mottled areas of T1 hypointensity
  - o Heterogeneous post-gadolinium enhancement
- Compression fractures of variable central canal narrowing

Bone Scan Findings
- Photopenic areas

Plain Film Findings
- Diffuse osteopenia (85%)
- Multiple, well-circumscribed, punched-out lesions (80%), may be expansile
- Approximately 1% of lesions are sclerotic
- Endosteal scalloping
- Soft-tissue mass adjacent to bone destruction
- Pathologic fractures
- Plasmacytoma: Solitary, large, expansile lesion (spine, pelvis, ribs), may be septated
- POEMS syndrome
  - o Enthesopathies of posterior elements of thoracic and lumbar spine
  - o Lytic lesions with surrounding sclerosis

Imaging Recommendations
- FSE T2 with fat saturation, STIR, or post-gadolinium T1WI increases the conspicuity of lesions

Differential Diagnosis

Metastases
- Pedicles involved first (late involvement in myeloma)
- Increased activity on bone scan

- Usually does **not** involve mandible

Severe Osteoporosis
- No endosteal scalloping on plain film
- Difficult to distinguish from diffuse marrow involvement on MRI

Pathology
General
- Etiology-Pathogenesis
  - Uncontrolled proliferation of plasma cells within bone marrow, secreting nonfunctional monoclonal immunoglobulins
- Epidemiology
  - Peak incidence from fourth to eighth decades of life with peak age at 64; rarely presents before 40 years of age
  - M: F = 3:2
  - 3 in 100,000 persons per year

Gross Pathologic-Surgical Features
- Confluent or well-circumscribed, red-gray, soft tumor replacing cancellous bone

Microscopic Features
- Aggregates of neoplastic plasma cells infiltrate and completely replace normal hematopoietic and fatty marrow
- Myeloma cells: Eccentric, round, hyperchromatic nuclei with "cartwheel" distribution of chromatin

Clinical Issues
Presentation
- Mild transient bone pain, worsened by activity (75%)
- Anemia, fever, weight loss
- Hypercalcemia
- Bence Jones proteins in urine
- Electrophoresis: Monoclonal gammopathy (IgA/ IgG peak)
- Pathologic fractures
- Amyloidosis (10%)

Treatment
- Radiation and chemotherapy
- Osteoclast inhibiting agents: Bisphosphates
- Vertebroplasty to stabilize vertebral bodies and relieve pain

Prognosis
- Survival time of 3 to 5 years with chemotherapy

Selected References
1. Lecouvet FE et al: Skeletal survey in advanced multiple myeloma: Radiographic versus MR imaging survey. Br J Haematol 106:35-9, 1999
2. Moulopoulos LA et al: Multiple myeloma: Spinal MR imaging in patients with untreated newly diagnosed disease. Radiology 185:833-40, 1992
3. Libshitz HI et al: Multiple myeloma: Appearance at MR imaging. Radiology 182:833-7, 1992

Paget Disease

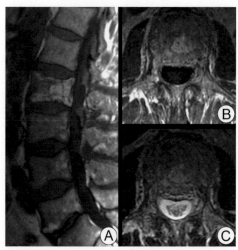

Sagittal T1WI of the lumbar spine (A) demonstrates an abnormal L2 vertebral body, slightly enlarged in the anterior-posterior dimension. Axial T1WI (B) and T2WI (C) reveal a diffusely coarsened and haphazard trabecular pattern.

Key Facts
- Synonym: Osteitis deformans
- Definition: Chronic disorder of abnormal bone remodeling in the adult skeleton
- Classic imaging appearance: "Picture frame" or "ivory" vertebra
- Vertebral involvement in 75% of patients with Paget disease
  - Most common in the lumbar spine (L3 and L4)
- Pelvis = spine > femur > skull > tibia > clavicle > humerus > ribs
- Monostotic or polyostotic, asymmetric
- Long bones: Lesion starts at one end of bone, extends along shaft
- Sarcomatous transformation (< 1%)
  - Osteosarcoma (22-90%)
  - Fibrosarcoma/MFH (29-51%)
  - Chondrosarcoma (1-15%)

Imaging Findings
General Features
- Best imaging clue: Enlarged vertebra with peripheral coarsening
Plain Film Findings
- Expanded and square vertebra
- Coarsened and dense peripheral trabecular pattern
- Relative lucent center
- Diffusely dense "ivory" vertebra
- Pathologic compression fracture
- Rarely solitary discrete lytic lesion
CT Findings
- Osseous enlargement
- Thickened cortex
- Coarsened trabeculae
- Dense enhancement in lytic phase

Paget Disease

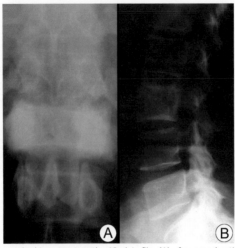

An "ivory" vertebral is present on the AP plain film (A) of a second patient. Lateral plain film (B) of a third patient shows a "picture frame" L3 vertebral body.

MR Findings
- Cortical thickening, increased size of bone, and coarse trabeculae
  - Pedicle, laminae, and spinal process also involved
- Dense bone hypointense on T1WI and T2WI
- Vascular marrow in active phase hyperintense on T2WI with fat saturation
  - May show postgadolinium enhancement on T1WI
- Variable degree of spinal stenosis

Tc-99m Diphosphonate Bone Scintigraphy Findings
- Increased uptake in lytic phase
- Normal scan in sclerotic, burned-out lesions
- Best modality in determining the extent of disease and monitoring disease response to medications

Differential Diagnosis
Osteoblastic Metastases
- More discrete
- May be hyperintense on FSE T2WI or STIR
- Lacks the "picture frame" appearance on plain film
- May be indistinguishable if "ivory" vertebra present

Hemangioma
- Typically hyperintense on T1WI and T2WI
- Stippled appearance on axial CT
- Striated appearance on plain film without vertebral enlargement

Pathology
General
- General Path Comments
  - Overactive osteoclasts and osteoblasts resulting in abnormal and disordered bone remodeling

Paget Disease

- Etiology-Pathogenesis
  - Familial incidence
  - Possible viral etiology
- Epidemiology
  - 3% of individuals over 40 years and 10% of those over 80 years
  - M: F = 3:2

Gross Pathologic-Surgical Features
- Newly formed bone abnormally enlarged, deformed, and softened

Microscopic Features
- Active phase (osteolytic phase)
  - Aggressive bone resorption with lytic lesions
  - Replacement of hematopoietic bone marrow by fibrous connective tissue
  - Increased vascular channels
- Inactive phase (quiescent phase)
  - Decreased bone turnover with skeletal sclerosis and coarse trabeculae
  - Loss of excessive vascularity
- Mixed pattern
  - Mixture of lytic and sclerotic phase

Clinical Issues

Presentation
- Age: 55-85 years, unusual <40 years
- Asymptomatic: 20%
- Deep, achy bone pain
- Spinal cord compression from vertebral enlargement or basilar invagination
- Pathologic fractures including vertebral collapse
- Sarcomatous transformation (< 1%)
- Elevated serum alkaline phosphatase and urine hydroxyproline

Treatment
- Analgesic medications
- Medicine to arrest osteoclastic activity
  - Bisphosphates: Alendronate, etidronate
  - Calcitonin
- Surgical decompression of spinal stenosis

Prognosis
- Disease process may be halted with possible return of normal osseous architecture with medications

Selected References
1. Boutin RD et al: Complications in Paget disease at MR imaging. Radiology 209:641-51, 1998
2. Roberts MC et al: Paget disease: MR imaging findings. Radiology 173:341-5, 1989
3. Frame B et al: Paget disease: A review of current knowledge. Radiology 141:21-4, 1981

Postirradiation Vertebral Marrow

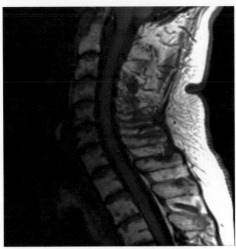

Sagittal T1WI of the cervical spine in a patient with multiple myeloma and previous radiation therapy demonstrates hyperintense marrow with scattered myelomatous foci.

Key Facts
- Definition: Fatty conversion of vertebral marrow after therapeutic irradiation
- Classic imaging appearance: Diffuse marrow hyperintensity corresponding to radiation portal on T1WI
- Dependent on
  - Radiation dose
  - Fractionation
  - Time elapsed
- No change in marrow signal intensity (SI) when radiation dose of 1.25 Gy was administered in one series
- At 50 Gy, persistent fat SI even after 9 years
  - Complete and irreversible eradication of cellular elements
- Between 20 to 30 Gy, return to normal marrow pattern after long-term follow-up (>10years)

Imaging Findings
General Features
- Best imaging clue: Marrow SI approaching that of subcutaneous fat on T1WI
CT Findings
- Diminished bone mass on dual energy CT study
- Compression fractures
MR Findings
- First three weeks
  - No change or early marrow T1 hyperintensity
  - Hyperintensity on STIR
    - Indicating marrow edema
    - Peak incidence nine days after irradiation
    - Subsequent gradual decrease in SI

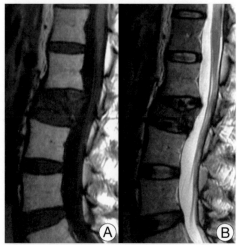

In a second patient who had a history of lumbar irradiation, sagittal T1WI (A) shows diffuse homogenous marrow hyperintensity, with the exception of L2 vertebral body, which is collapsed and hypointense on T1WI and T2WI (B). The fatty vertebral marrow demonstrates intermediate signal intensity on T2WI (B).

- Three to six weeks
  - Heterogeneous mottled pattern on T1WI, or
  - Increasing fat intensity within the central vertebral marrow
    - Surrounding the basivertebral vein
- After six weeks
  - Diffuse and homogenous hyperintensity on T1WI, or
  - Band pattern of peripheral intermediate SI
    - Surrounding central hyperintense marrow
    - May represent regenerating hematopoietic marrow

Nuclear Medicine Findings
- Focal or diffuse diminished radio-tracer uptake on Tc-99m diphosphonate and Tc-99m sulfur colloid scans
  - Corresponding to radiation portal

Imaging Recommendations
- STIR or FSE T2WI with fat saturation to better assess recurrent or residual marrow disease
- Pre- and postgadolinium T1WI with fat saturation also increases lesion conspicuity

Differential Diagnosis

Focal Marrow Infarction
- Serpiginous border between normal and infarcted marrow
  - Hyperintense on STIR or FSE T2WI with fat saturation
  - Surrounding marrow edema
  - May enhance after intravenous gadolinium
- May be difficult to distinguish from recurrent metastasis
  - Biopsy indicated

Postirradiation Vertebral Marrow

Pathology
General
- General Path Comments
  - Radiation destroys hematopoietic marrow elements
  - Reduction of bone mass also occurs
  - Fatty marrow replacement of celluar marrow and bone loss

Microscopic Features
- Based on rat model after single dose of irradiation at 20 Gy
- Initially decreased cellular elements and disrupted sinusoids
  - Associated edema and hemorrhage
- Early influx of cells to re-populate the marrow
  - Concomitant increase in fatty marrow
- Subsequent depletion of cellularity and sinusoids
  - Fibrosis with increasing fatty marrow
- Eventual regeneration of hematopoietic elements and sinusoids

Clinical Issues
Presentation
- Usually asymptomatic
- Pain related to radiation necrosis or
- Insufficiency fracture from weakened bone

Natural History
- Return to normal marrow pattern on long-term follow-up

Treatment
- Supportive measures

Prognosis
- Dependent on underlying disease for which radiation therapy is employed

Selected References
1. Steiner RM et al: Magnetic resonance imaging of diffuse bone marrow disease. Radiol Clin of North Am 31:383-409, 1993
2. Yankelevitz DF et al: Effect of radiation therapy on thoracic and lumbar bone marrow: Evaluation with MR imaging. AJR 157:87-92, 1991
3. Stevens SK et al: Early and late bone-marrow changes after irradiation: MR evaluation. AJR 154:745-50, 1990

PERIPHERAL NERVE PLEXUS IMAGING

Brachial Plexus Avulsion

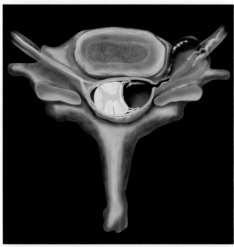

Nerve root avulsion. Drawing depicts avulsion of a left cervical nerve root at its junction with the cervical cord. There is also a dural laceration with pseudomeningocele formation compressing the cervical spinal cord.

Key Facts
- Synonym: Cervical pseudomeningocele(s)
- Definition: Avulsion of one or more cervical root components of the brachial plexus (C5–T1) from the spinal cord
- Classic imaging appearance: Lateral thecal sac outpouchings (diverticula); devoid of neural elements
- Clinical sensory and motor deficits reflect roots involved

Imaging Findings
General Features
- Best imaging clue: CSF filled outpouchings of lateral thecal sac
CT Findings
- Difficult diagnosis on unenhanced CT; may see pseudomeningocele(s)
- Look for hematoma in paraspinal tissues or scalene muscles
- CT myelography shows dilated empty root sleeves, CSF leak in rare cases
MR Findings
- Dilated CSF signal intensity within empty thecal sac diverticulum
- May see associated spinal cord abnormality
- Search for signs of soft tissue trauma (edema, hemorrhage) or fracture
- Characteristic findings on high resolution MR imaging ("MR neurography")
  - Attenuated or disrupted proximal roots/rami within or immediately distal to diverticulum
  - Swollen and retracted distal nerve roots
  - Nerve "retraction ball"
Other Modality Findings
- Plain films rarely helpful
Imaging Recommendations
- Conventional CT is of limited utility

Brachial Plexus Avulsion

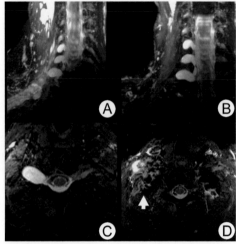

(A, B) Coronal MPR FSEIR sequence shows C5, C6, and C7 pseudomeningoceles transection of the proximal nerve roots, which have retracted into a "ball", and swollen distal plexus. (C, D) Axial FSEIR images show pseudomeningoceles and retracted avulsed plexus elements (arrow).

- High resolution MR "neurographic" imaging technique best demonstrates plexus architecture and injury extent
  - Coronal T1WI and FSEIR, oblique sagittal T1WI and FSEIR sequences
  - CT myelography if MR contraindications or MRI is inconclusive

Differential Diagnosis
Nerve Sheath Tumor
- Plexiform neurofibroma (Neurofibromatosis type 1; NF-1) or solitary nerve sheath tumor mimics root avulsion(s)
- Search for clinical or imaging stigmata of NF-1 or trauma to differentiate
Dural Dysplasia
- Marfan's syndrome, Ehlers-Danlos syndrome, NF-1)
- Lateral meningocele(s) mimic pseudomeningocele
- Clinical stigmata, dural dysplasia distinguish from trauma
Nerve Root Sleeve Cyst
- Usually asymptomatic incidental finding; may be quite large
- Spontaneous rupture may present with intracranial hypotension
- Appropriate clinical history helps distinguish from avulsion

Pathology
General
- General Path Comments
  - Traction on brachial plexus avulses one or more nerve roots from the spinal cord at root entry zone
  - Neurological deficits can be partially predicted from injured roots
  - However, many muscles receive innervation from multiple roots
    - Not uncommon to see incomplete paralysis in patients with complete root avulsion(s)

Brachial Plexus Avulsion

- Anatomy
  - Brachial plexus normally composed of C5, C6, C7, C8, and T1 roots
  - Roots coalesce to sequentially form rami, trunks, divisions, trunks, and peripheral branches (proximal to distal)
- Etiology-Pathogenesis
  - May result from either penetrating or blunt traction injury

Gross Pathologic-Surgical Features
- Familiarity with normal brachial plexus anatomy essential for MR imaging interpretation
- Integrity of questioned nerve roots critical for surgical decision making
  - Stretched but contiguous nerves may recover some function
  - Completely avulsed nerve roots produce irreversible sensory and motor deficits

Clinical Issues
Presentation
- Brachial plexus syndromes reflect functional loss in territory of avulsed root(s)
  - Nevertheless, partial paralysis and incomplete sensory loss are common because innervation is redundant
- Complete brachial plexus avulsion produces useless "flail arm"
- Incomplete injuries produce isolated radiculopathy or classic syndrome
  - Erb-Duchenne palsy
    - Upper plexus injury (C5, C6 roots, upper trunk)
    - Proximal muscle weakness
    - Direct blow to shoulder, birth traction injury
  - Middle radicular syndrome
    - C7 root, middle trunk – findings primarily in radial nerve territory
  - Klumpke palsy
    - Lower plexus injury (C8, T1 roots, lower trunk)
    - Distal muscle weakness

Treatment
- Conservative rehabilitation management
- Re-anastomosis of avulsed roots to spinal cord not generally advocated
  - New microsurgical techniques prompting re-review
- Amputation in selected cases of "flail arm"

Prognosis
- Variable but generally poor

Selected References
1. Terzis JK et al: Brachial plexus root avulsions. World J Surg 25(8): 1049-61, 2001
2. Aagaard BD et al: Magnetic resonance neurography: magnetic resonance imaging of peripheral nerves. Neuroimaging Clin N Am 11(1): 131-46, 2001
3. Rowland L: Merritt's textbook of neurology. Eighth ed., Lea & Febiger: Philadelphia, 1989

Brachial Plexus Neuroma

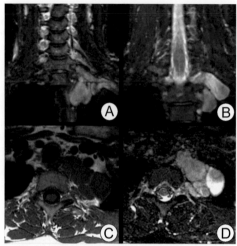

NF-1. (A, B) Coronal FSEIR images show abnormal enlargement and T2 hyperintensity of the left C8 and T1 rami extending into the lower trunk. (C, D) Axial T1 and FSEIR images confirm enlarged left lower trunk with classic hypointense T1 and hyperintense T2 appearance.

Key Facts
- Synonym(s): Brachial plexus neurofibroma or schwannoma
- Definition: Nerve sheath tumor arising within brachial plexus
- Classic imaging appearance: Fusiform, lobulated mass in the course of the plexus elements
- Plexiform neurofibroma in neurofibromatosis type 1 (NF-1) patient most common- may be infiltrative rather than masslike
  - Less commonly schwannoma in patient with NF-2
  - Isolated plexus schwannoma or neurofibroma less common

Imaging Findings
General Features
- Normal nerve is hypo- to isointense (to muscle) on T1WI, mildly hyperintense on T2WI
  - Compared to normal nerve and muscle, nerve sheath tumors are abnormally bright on T2WI and enhance with contrast
- Best imaging clue: Lobulated mass with abnormal T2 hyperintensity and contrast enhancement
CT Findings
- Fusiform enlargement of plexus components and distortion of normal regional soft-tissue architecture
  - Much more difficult to appreciate on CT than MR imaging
  - Osseous foraminal enlargement, dural ectasia variable
MR Findings
- Fusiform brachial plexus enlargement and abnormal T2 hyperintensity (approaching signal of regional vessels)
- Moderate to avid enhancement compared with normal nerves
Imaging Recommendations
- CT is of limited utility

Brachial Plexus Neuroma

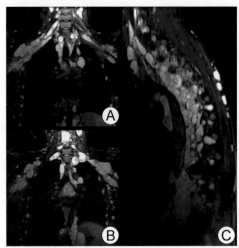

NF-1. (A, B) Coronal FSEIR images show extensive bilateral involvement of the brachial plexus. Note also numerous paraspinal neurofibromas. (C) Sagittal FSIER image confirms abnormal lower cervical rami and further demonstrates extensive paraspinal neurofibromas.

- High resolution MR "neurographic" imaging technique best demonstrates plexus architecture and disease extent
  - Coronal T1 and FSEIR, oblique sagittal T1 and FSEIR, coronal and oblique sagittal contrast-enhanced fat-saturated T1 sequences

Differential Diagnosis
Chronic inflammatory Demyelinating Polyneuropathy (CIDP)
- Inflammatory peripheral polyneuropathy
- Clinical and laboratory profile differs from NF-1
Inherited Demyelinating Polyneuropathy (Charcot-Marie-Tooth, Dejerine-Sottas Disease)
- Genetic testing and clinical phenotype help distinguish from NF-1
Metastatic Tumor
- Mass with local soft tissue invasion; appropriate clinical history
Pseudomeningocele
- CSF signal
- More spherical/ovoid

Pathology
General
- General Path Comments
  - World Health Organization (WHO) criteria for NF-1 and NF-2
    - NF-1: Multiple neurofibromas, optic nerve gliomas and other astrocytomas, café-au-lait spots, axillary freckling, and iris hamartomas
    - NF-2: Multiple schwannomas, ependymomas, and meningiomas
- Genetics
  - NF-1: Autosomal dominant, gene locus on chromosome 17q12
  - NF-2: Autosomal dominant, gene locus on chromosome 22q12

- o Isolated nerve sheath tumors are usually not inherited
- Epidemiology
  - o Prevalence of NF-1 1:4000; 50% new mutations
  - o Prevalence of NF-2 1:40,000; 50% new mutations

Gross Pathologic-Surgical Features

- Neurofibromas and schwannomas are benign (WHO grade I)
  - o Both are firm, well-circumscribed, gray-tan, fusiform masses
  - o Plexiform neurofibromas resemble a bag of worms
- Plexiform neurofibromas and neurofibromas of large nerves are postulated to be the precursor of most malignant peripheral nerve sheath tumors (MPNSTs)

Microscopic Features

- Neurofibroma: Neoplastic Schwann cells, perineural-like cells, and fibroblasts within a collagen matrix
  - o Axons are usually imbedded within tumor
- Schwannoma: Neoplastic Schwann cells
  - o More frequently located peripheral to axons
  - o Often shows cysts and hemorrhage
  - o Proportion of two characteristic architectures (Antoni A and B patterns) determines gross appearance

Clinical Issues

Presentation

- Asymptomatic, palpable mass, radiculopathy, or peripheral neuropathy
- Pain is worrisome feature that may indicate malignant transformation

Natural History

- Slow growing benign tumors
- Development of pain may indicate malignant transformation

Treatment

- Solitary tumors often resectable
  - o May require nerve sacrifice
- Diffuse lesions are generally unresectable

Prognosis

- Frequently asymptomatic or palpable nuisance only
- Malignant transformation to MPNST has poor prognosis

Selected References
1. Kleihues P et al: Pathology and genetics of tumours of the nervous system. Lyon: IARC Press, 2000
2. Maravilla K et al: Imaging of the peripheral nervous system: evaluation of peripheral neuropathy and plexopathy. Am J Neuroradiol 19: 1011-23, 1998
3. Filler AG et al: Application of magnetic resonance neurography in the evaluation of patients with peripheral nerve pathology. J Neurosurg 85(2): 299-309, 1996

Radiation Plexopathy

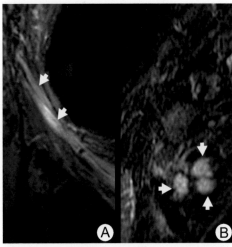

Radiation Plexopathy. (A) Coronal FSIER shows diffuse enlargement and hyperintensity of the upper plexus (arrows). (B) Oblique sagittal FSIER confirms diffuse enlargement of the cords (arrows).

Key Facts
- Definition: Radiation induced nerve brachial plexus injury
- Classic imaging appearance
  - Diffuse plexus enlargement with relatively homogeneous T2 hyperintensity of multiple components
  - Frequently homogeneous enhancement
  - Usually involves upper brachial plexus (C5, 6, 7)
- Similar to lumbosacral plexopathy following pelvic irradiation
- Uncommon below 60 Gray dose
  - Dose-dependant; potentiated by chemotherapy
  - Rare (< 1% incidence)
  - Delayed onset (5-30 months post-therapy)

Imaging Findings
General Features
- Best imaging clue: Smooth, diffuse T2 hyperintensity of multiple trunks or divisions (especially upper brachial plexus)
CT Findings
- Diffuse plexus enlargement – very difficult CT diagnosis
MR Findings
- T1WI – diffuse nerve enlargement with mild hypointensity; diffuse enhancement without focal nodularity
- T2WI – Diffuse hyperintensity maintains plexus architecture
Imaging Recommendations
- Coronal and oblique sagittal best imaging planes
- Fat suppression essential on T2 weighted and gadolinium enhanced sequences

Radiation Plexopathy

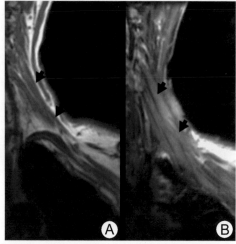

Radiation plexopathy. (A) Coronal T1WI shows diffuse enlargement and hypointensity of the upper plexus (arrows). No focal nodularity or adjacent adenopathy. (B) Coronal T1WI with contrast confirms characteristic homogeneous diffuse plexus enhancement (arrows).

Differential Diagnosis
Malignant Brachial Plexus Infiltration
- Most commonly involves the inferior brachial plexus (C7, C8, T1)
- Direct extension from axillary adenopathy (breast cancer) or lung apex (Pancoast tumor)
- More focal and nodular than radiation plexopathy

Pathology
General
- Pathogenesis is poorly understood
- Etiology-Pathogenesis
  - Combination of direct cell damage from ionizing radiation and progressive ischemia
Gross Pathologic-Surgical Features
- Characterized by gross tissue atrophy and fibrosis
  - Fibrous thickening of nerve sheath
  - Demyelination
  - Fibrous replacement of nerve fibers

Clinical Issues
Presentation
- Pain and sensory loss in affected limb followed by motor strength loss
- Usually referable to upper brachial plexus (C5, 6, 7)
- Horner syndrome rare
- Delayed onset – usually 10 to 20 months post-treatment
Treatment
- Conservative – corticosteroids may help
- Avoid additional radiation

Radiation Plexopathy

<u>Prognosis</u>
- Variable

Selected References
1. Cros D: Peripheral Neuropathy. First ed, Philadelphia: Lippincott Williams & Wilkins. 185-7, 2001
2. Qayyum A et al: Symptomatic brachial plexopathy following treatment for breast cancer: utility of MR imaging with surface-coil techniques. Radiology 214(3): 837-42, 2000
3. Bowen BC et al: Radiation-induced brachial plexopathy: MR and clinical findings. AJNR 17(10): 1932-6, 1996

Index of Diagnoses